LUPUS
The Battle Within

A Woman's Most Intimate Life Story

VALERIE HORN

VJH
Publishing
Atlanta, Georgia

LUPUS: The Battle Within

A Woman's Most Intimate Life Story

Copyright © 2016 by Valerie Horn

Editor: Courtney Lindemann

Art Direction, Design, Cover Art, Interior Art: Christopher Bethune

First Edition

Published by VJH Publishing
Atlanta, Georgia
www.valeriehorn.com

ISBN-13: 978-0692692806
ISBN-10: 0692692800

Printed in the United States of America

If you liked this book, let others know.
Connect with the author at: www.valeriehorn.com

DEDICATION

This book is dedicated to my three children, Christine, Christopher, and Christel, who have been there through good times and bad.

To my mother, Lillian Colley, and my stepfather, Major Colley, Sr., who were the guiding force in my life, who gave their unconditional love and support.

To the doctors who have helped me, and especially to Dr. Christine Lawrence, who I named my oldest daughter after, who was a compassionate and caring doctor, who dedicated a portion of her life to helping patients with lupus.

To Dr. Betty Diamond, who I also named my youngest daughter after, who was also a compassionate and caring doctor who continues to study lupus, including the cognitive problems patients often experience, and to try to develop new, less toxic therapies for Systemic Lupus Erythematosus (SLE).

✦ CONTENTS ✦

CONTENTS

PREFACE

I would first like to take a moment and say that this has certainly been a time to remember and I never thought it could happen to me.

Since I was very young, I began writing about my life living with lupus. I documented each stage of my life because I wanted the world to know what I was going through. I always kept the two stenography books that I had been writing in inside my night table. I felt that if one day I really got sick, or even died, maybe someone would just go to my night table, pull out the drawer, and pick up those two stenography books. Maybe they would read Part I and Part II and see all the challenges that I had to face. I thank God for giving me the wisdom, the guidance, and the strength to continue writing my story.

Why Did I Decide to Write a Book?

On July 30, 2012, I was sitting at the kitchen table when my oldest daughter, Christine, had just come in from a busy day at work. My daughter, looked at me with excitement and said, "Mom, you know those two steno notebooks that you always keep in your night table?" I said, "Yes." My daughter said, "You have been writing about lupus since you were very young. Mom, why don't you write a book?" I said, "A book!" She said, "Yes." She told me that my book could help a lot of people who are also dealing with the same disease. She said, "Mom, let this book be your legacy, detailing the challenges you had to face. You have a story to tell!" That was all I needed to hear. When my daughter used the word legacy, I do not know what happened! It was not the word "book" that did it for me, but the word "legacy." It gave me a feeling inside that I could not even explain. I said, "Okay, Christine that will not be a problem for me; especially since none of you have ever read my story."

I walked up the stairs to my bedroom and took out my two stenography notebooks that I had been writing in for so long. I was so excited that I called my doctor at her home in New York City. She was so glad to hear my voice. I told her that Christine was encouraging me to write my "lupus story" and the challenges I had to face. She was very happy to hear what I was planning on doing. I have had this doctor since a very young age—from when I was first diagnosed with lupus—and I have never lost contact with her. I asked her if there was anything concerning her that she would like me to include in my book. She told me to write whatever I wanted to write about and that it would not be a problem for her. She said, "All I ask is that you do one thing for me, Valerie." I said, "What is that?" She said, "Can you please have your son be the illustrator of your book?" I said, "Sure, that is what I already planned on doing." Dr. Lawrence already knew that my son, Christopher, was in college at the time and was pursuing a career in illustration and design. My doctor was so pleased to hear that, and I was very happy to hear her ask that of me.

So, with that in mind, I sat in front of my computer and started reminiscing about the life I've lived and the memories I've created. Heavily engrossed in writing my lupus story, it has been a labor of love and I hope that it brings peace to everyone that reads it.

LUPUS
The Battle Within

PART I

CHILDHOOD
INTO
ADULTHOOD

CHAPTER 1

MY STORY BEGINS

My name is Valerie Jean Blackwood. I was born on June 27, 1952, in Lincoln Hospital, in the Bronx, New York, to the parents of Lillian and Arthur Blackwood. My mother was born in Bermuda, and my father was born in the British West Indies. I was baptized on December 14, 1952.

When I was five years old, my family and I lived in the Bronx, New York, in the housing projects known as Throggs Neck. My mother and father were separated.

One day, my father came over to visit us. We were on our way to the store when I saw some children playing and running around outside. They were having so much fun that they bumped into me, while my father and I were walking on the sidewalk and I fell to the ground. I felt at least two of the children step on my little right pinky finger. When I managed to get up from the sidewalk, I was hysterical and holding my hand closed with my finger throbbing. I told my father that my finger was really hurting me. On our way home, my father took a look at it and said, "Don't say a word to nobody." My father knew that my mother would have been livid at him for not even holding my hand while we were outside. So, with that secret in mind, my finger stayed broken.

A Certificate of Promotion

On June 22, 1958, I received a Certificate of Promotion from the Kindergarten Department to the Primary Department of the Fort Schuyler Presbyterian Church, where I was attending. I was six years old when my father passed away at the age of forty-five.

Elementary School

Second Grade

When I was in the second grade, during September 1959 to June 1960, I attended P.S. 72, in the Bronx, New York. My teacher, Mrs. Quinn, gave me a report that showed how I got along in school and my growth as a child. She stated: "Valerie is a well-behaved child. She gets along well with the other children. She does her work conscientiously to satisfaction. Her written work has been posted on the bulletin board. She reads on grade level and can answer questions on what she has read. She gets 100% in spelling and can apply her words in written expression. She does not volunteer as much as she should in class discussion. Her written expression shows originality. She understands mathematics and knows her number stories. She likes to paint. She does well in arts and crafts. Valerie is a quiet child. She enjoys playing with the other children. She should take a more active part. She does her work carefully. She finishes promptly and is accurate. She observes health and safety rules."

My feelings as a child in second grade

At that young stage in my life, I enjoyed going to school each and every day. I loved the feeling it gave me inside when I was able to write in class, as well as learn new words. One thing that Mrs. Quinn did to make spelling fun, was pick words from our homework assignments and then break us up into teams. She would point to each person from the team, and we would have to say the words aloud. Whichever team was not able to spell the words correctly, would have to sit down. The team left standing after all of the words were called was the winner.

Arts and crafts was also something that I really enjoyed. I was always happy and ready to paint and do all of the fun things that my teacher instructed us to do. In class, I was a very quiet child, but I enjoyed being around the other children. I was so focused and wanted to do all of my work carefully. I also enjoyed going to Sunday school at the Fort Schuyler Presbyterian Church.

Third Grade

I was in the third grade from September 1960 to June 1961. I was in a new school called P.S. 71. The report I received from my teacher, Mrs. Dursi, showed how

I got along in school and my growth as a child. She stated: "Valerie always obeys the rules for good conduct. She does not finish her work fast enough. She begins promptly, but needs to work faster. Valerie reads well on the third grade level. She must learn to speak louder. Valerie does well in spelling and penmanship. She can try harder with her math. Valerie is very much interested in arts and crafts. Valerie accepts good standards of conduct. She writes well and her spelling is very good."

My feelings as a child in third grade

When I was in third grade, I tried so hard to make my work look perfect, so I took my time and wrote very slowly. But, some of the other children would always finish before me. I was so shy and quiet that I did not like it when I was called upon to speak aloud in class. Also, math for me was a little challenging.

Fourth Grade

When I was in the fourth grade, from September 1961 to June 1962, the report that I received from my teacher, Ms. Ciminello, showed how I got along in school and my growth as a child. Ms. Ciminello stated: "Valerie is a very polite child. She always wants to help. She shows initiative. Her work is carefully done. She enjoys reading and has very little difficulty attacking new words. She moves from one idea to another in smooth transition. She has original ideas and presents them in a neat and clear fashion. She has developed skill and accuracy. Valerie is eager to cooperate and willing to help. She takes great pride in her work. She is able to follow plot development and story design. Valerie has acquired automatic mastery of words frequently written and needed in other content areas."

My feelings as a child in fourth grade

Ms. Ciminello was very nice. I enjoyed being in her class so much. She made the work so easy for me to understand. The funny thing about it was, she was a tough teacher, and yet I looked forward to being in her class. Being such a quiet child, she really brought out the very best in me.

Fifth Grade

I was in the fifth grade from September 1962 to June 1963. I received a report from my teacher, Ms. Leitman, that showed how I was getting along in school and my growth as a child. Ms. Leitman stated: "Valerie is attentive and well maintained. Let us try to encourage her to be more outgoing. Valerie works carefully and usually completes every job. She is thorough in all her work and is very conscientious about finishing her assigned tasks. Valerie's handwriting is lovely. She does very well in spelling. She is able to sound out new words, but does not always understand everything that she reads. In math, she needs help understanding fractions and long division."

My feelings as a child in fifth grade

School started during September 1962. My mother got remarried two months into the school year, on November 10, 1962. My new dad, Major Colley Sr., had three children of his own. He had two sons and one daughter (Alonzo, Etta Mae, and his youngest son, Major Jr., named after my stepfather). My mother had four children of her own. She had one son and three daughters (Reginald, Vanessa, Claudette, and I was the middle child).

During that time, I started showing a lot more improvement. I started speaking more loudly and clearly in class. Ms. Leitman was the kind of teacher that did not like it if you were a little too quiet, and that was definitely me. When I would finish my social studies reports in a relatively fast manner, then present it to her before it was due, she would turn around and give me some extra reports for homework to do. Then, after doing all of those long assignments, she would turn around and give me a "Fair" for a grade. I couldn't believe what she was doing to me! My mother had to write a letter to Ms. Leitman stating: "Please do not give my daughter any more extra work to do if she is going to get marks like this! If she is smart enough to do the work, then she should receive a decent mark." After that letter was put on her desk, Ms. Leitman asked the class, "Whose mother's name is "Lillian Colley?" I was just quietly sitting in the class; the name did not even register at all. My cousin, Pat, who was also in the same class with me, said,

"Valerie, isn't that your mother's married name." I was very embarrassed as I raised my hand. I thought to myself, *"Leave it to my cousin to remember my mother's married name."*

Soon after my mother was married, we became a family of nine, and we could no longer live in the Throggs Neck housing projects that my mother loved so much. They were able to find a brand new development in the Bronx, with a much larger apartment that accommodated all of us. The apartment was very pretty and very big, and it even had two bathrooms. But, after moving in, my mother was not happy with where we were living. So, they decided that they would not stay there too long. Their primary goal was to purchase a home of their own.

Sixth Grade

My feelings as a child in a New Neighborhood/New School in the Bronx, New York

With hard work and determination on my parent's part, in less than a year, they purchased their own home. It was an older home that needed some work, but in due time, my stepfather, who I call my father, said he would take care of it. My siblings and I were not too happy about the quick move. We had made so many new friends and school was almost ending. The new neighborhood was so different. It was extremely quiet and something that we had to get used to.

During the springtime of 1964, my mother entered me into P.S. 41, where I began the latter part of my sixth grade school year. I did not like walking to school all by myself and that was a period of adjustment for me. My siblings were older, so they were in a different school. I was glad that I did not have too much longer before I could go to that new school as well, and I wished that the time would just hurry up! For the short time that I was in P.S. 41, I noticed that their academics were so much more advanced than where I was before. Mrs. Levine had to look up my grades from the old school in order to make a determination of whether or not I would be able to graduate with the sixth grade class and move on to junior high school.

After looking over my previous school records, Mrs. Levine said that it would not be fair to keep me back. She told my mother that, due to the fact that my school records showed I was doing well in fifth grade, I would be able to graduate. I was so happy that everything worked out well for me. I was able to graduate in my white flowered dress, but not at all happy to be wearing those white 'bobby socks' that my mother had me wear on my special day.

Being able to graduate filled me with so much pride. I looked forward to having a very happy and beautiful summer vacation, as I prepared to enter the seventh grade in yet another new school come September.

Junior High School

Seventh Grade

During the fall of 1964, I was attending Junior High School 113. I was twelve years old by the time I was finally in the same school as some of my siblings. After getting situated in school, something different was starting to happen to me, but I did not know what it was. Some days, I just didn't feel well. My grades even began to drop tremendously. I was just lagging behind and struggling in school. My strength was always in Language Arts and Spelling. That was major for me. It really helped me out a lot when my other subjects were lacking. On May 27, 1965, I received from my seventh grade teacher, a Commendation Card award for excellence in spelling. I was happy because I knew the struggle I had been going through. With determination and hard work, I made it through that school year. I was able to move on to the eighth grade.

Explaining What Happened to My Finger

During my summer vacation that year, I had time to relax, have fun, and be with my family. One day, when my family and I were sitting down at the dining room table, my stepfather noticed that my right pinky finger was not straight.

"Valerie, can you straighten out your pinky?" He asked.

"No." I answered.

"Let me see your finger?" My mother said, coming over to me. "What happened to your finger?"

"It's broken." I said, matter-of-factly.

"Broken?" she exclaimed.

"Yes, Mommy."

"When did that happen?" She asked. I explained that it happened back when I was five years old—that my father had taken me to the store and some children were running around and playing as we were walking. I told her that they bumped into me, I fell to the ground, and they stepped on my finger—breaking it. I told my mother that it was so painful that I just always kept my finger closed.

My mother was so hurt that she found all this out after my biological father had died. She could not believe that he did not hold my hand at all as we walked together outside; especially because I was so young.

Soon after, my parents took me to Jacobi Hospital to see what could be done. As the doctors were looking at my pinky, they said too many years had gone by and that they would have to remove the bone in my finger. I would be left with a shorter pinky finger on that hand. That was really a disappointment to hear.

Because I was not comfortable having them remove the bone, the doctors decided that it was best to simply leave the finger the way it was, unless I was planning on doing hand commercials. I assured them I was not. So, my parents agreed to just leave the finger alone.

Eighth Grade

Before I knew it, the summer was already over and school started in September 1965. The struggles that I seemed to be experiencing in the seventh grade school year were so much better after I entered into the eighth grade. My grades were excellent. There is nothing more I can say about that school year. I just made sure that I continued to look forward to another good year.

Ninth Grade

At Prospect Medical Clinic – Fourteen Years Old

It was wintertime in 1966 and I was fourteen years old. I did not know what was happening to me. I woke up one morning and I could barely walk. After my mother saw my condition, she decided to take me to Prospect Medical Clinic, in the Bronx, New York.

Kidney Infection

When we arrived at the clinic, I had to give some urine. The test showed that I had a kidney infection. The doctor instructed me to start drinking plenty of water. Water was something that I did not like to drink a lot of, but I had to start. The doctor gave me some small brown vitamins to take when I got home. After about two weeks, I felt much better. For further observation, Prospect Medical Clinic referred me to Mount Sinai Hospital.

My Confirmation at St. Luke's Episcopal Church

When I attended St. Luke's Episcopal Church, I continued to socialize as much as I could by staying involved in all of the church activities. My siblings and I received our Confirmation from St. Luke's Episcopal Church on November 27, 1966. There were pictures taken at my parent's house on that special occasion.

Admitted to Mount Sinai Hospital in New York City

When I was in ninth grade, I noticed some lumps behind my ears. My family began to worry, even though those lumps did not hurt me at all. It was a cold and blustery day when my mother and father decided to take me to Mount Sinai Hospital. After being seen, the hospital decided that it would be best if I were admitted for further testing.

Biopsy of the Liver

After a short time had passed, my parents were informed that a biopsy of my liver should be taken. With my parent's approval, the biopsy was done as a bedside procedure, right in the same room I slept in, and not in the operating room. I was told to lie down on my side, so the doctor could find the correct spot. Then, that area was deadened. There was a very long, straight needle with a round hook at the end of it. That long needle was inserted into the area the doctor had prepped. When the needle was being pulled out, I saw that a piece of my liver had come out on the bottom of the hook.

Biopsy of the Skin

In addition to the strange bumps behind my ears, I was also having other troubles with my skin. My cheeks had a terrible rash. The rash started out red and then turned black. When I would wash my face, it burned dreadfully. My parents were informed that I would have to have another procedure done. So, with their approval, I had a biopsy of the skin.

For that procedure, I had to be in the operating room. After I was prepped for surgery, they explained that they would be taking a piece of skin from my face above my eyebrows on the left side. I then received anesthesia that allowed me to sleep through the process.

As I awoke, I was glad that my surgery was over. After spending a considerable amount of time in the hospital, they still could not find anything wrong with me. So, the hospital decided to discharge me. They did not administer any medications for me to take at home. My parents were told that I could continue to be seen as an outpatient.

Mount Sinai Hospital treated me so well for the month that I stayed there. Their food was excellent and I mean excellent! It was such a shame because I was too sick to even enjoy the beautiful meals that I was receiving. My weight was about 108 to 110 pounds.

I was so glad to be back at home with my family. But, I was definitely not looking forward to catching up on all of the schoolwork that I had missed.

When I returned back to school, it was so hard on me.

With a lot of determination and hard work, I was able to make it through to the end of my ninth grade school year. On June 27, 1967, I was able to graduate from junior high school. I received my Certificate of Completion for my ninth year course of study, along with my diploma. Although school was out for the summer, I was anxious to see how I would do in high school. My dream was to become a secretary.

High School

Tenth Grade

When my tenth grade school year started in September, I was advised that for the next three years, the secretarial courses that I needed to complete would include: English, American Studies, Biology, Stenography/Transcribing, Typing, Business Law, Bookkeeping, Economics, Hygiene, Health Education, Art, Music, and Gym, which also included Folk Dancing. The curriculum also required me to take swimming in order to graduate from Evander Childs High School. The two main classes that I was looking forward to taking were definitely Stenography and Typing.

After I took one of the main classes, I received no less than 90% in Typing. I still did not receive Stenography because I was told that the class was full. Therefore, my mother had to come to school and speak with my guidance counselor on that matter. It was not very easy. Through much persistence and determination, on my mother's part, I was able to receive that most important class for my career.

My Big Achievement

It was almost the end of the school year. As I was quietly sitting in class, my stenography teacher, Ms. Hicks, suddenly stood up by her desk. In front of the class, she made an announcement. "Excuse me class." She began, "You have all taken your final exam for Stenography 1. I would like to tell you that the student who has obtained the highest average of all the tenth grade classes is Valerie Blackwood." I was so shocked, excited, and proud of myself. I couldn't stop smiling!

Ms. Hicks continued, "Valerie has earned a 104%! Remember class, you were given an extra bonus of 4 points if you were able to transcribe something that you have not yet learned in this class. Valerie was able to transcribe material that will be taught in the eleventh grade class. I also want to point out to you, class, that since I believe no one is perfect…" she paused briefly as she looked directly at me. "Valerie, you will be receiving a 99% as a final grade in this class on your report card." On June 14, 1968, I was awarded a Certificate of Achievement from my teacher for having attained the highest standing of all classes for the term in Stenography 1. I also received a 100% on my final exam in Typing. I was ecstatic that I did so well and ended the school year beautifully. I did not let my health get the best of me, and I accomplished what I set out to do. I was able to enjoy a very nice summer vacation.

Eleventh Grade

I could not believe it. School just seemed to roll around again so quickly, and I had already started the eleventh grade school year.

Irregular Periods

When I was sixteen years old, I started experiencing irregular periods. Instead of monthly, it had been coming about every two to three months and lasted about a week. Luckily, I did not experience any pain, heavy bleeding, or discomfort during my periods.

Unbearable Body Aches

As the year progressed, I suddenly was beginning to feel like I didn't know what was happening to me again. I was experiencing tremendous pain in my bones and joints. My whole entire body simply ached. I knew that something had to be done quickly! I could not stand the excruciating pain anymore! All I could do was cry because the pain was unbearable. Time could not wait anymore, so my parents immediately took me to Jacobi Hospital in the Bronx, New York.

Admitted to Jacobi Hospital, Bronx, New York

When we arrived at Jacobi hospital and the doctors saw the excruciating pain I was in, they immediately decided that I should be admitted for further testing.

Bone Marrow Test

After being admitted, the doctors seemed to be taking blood from me all day and night. I felt that my skinny little arms could not take it anymore! My parents were informed by the doctors that they would be conducting a Bone Marrow Test on me. Fortunately, this was another bedside procedure, so I didn't have to deal with the added stress of surgery. The doctor explained that they would be inserting a needle straight into my bone and a syringe would be pulling out some fluid.

So, with my parent's approval, I was able to have the procedure done. The process was so painful that I could not prevent myself from screaming out loud. After it was done, all I could hope was that I would never, ever, have to go through that again. I was pleased to hear that the results from my Bone Marrow test were negative. That was a big relief. My urine tests were fairly normal as well.

After all the time I spent suffering through my illness, the doctors finally suggested that what I was experiencing was Arthritis.

"Arthritis…with all that my daughter has been going through, it doesn't sound like Arthritis to me!" My mother shouted. She was angry with the doctor's diagnosis because I was still not well at all. I was unable to eat and my head would ache something terrible. Yet, the true problem still remained a mystery!

Lymph Node Procedure

I was having an ongoing occurrence of lymph nodes

popping up behind my ears. After the doctors saw what was happening, they requested that another procedure be done. The procedure required taking a piece of lymph node out from behind my ear, so that they could test the tissue and see what was going on with me. So, with my parent's approval, I would have yet another procedure done. I was really scared. For one so young, I had already gone through so much and I had suffered through turmoil for far too long. I prayed that when the operation was over, the doctors would finally have the answers to all of our questions.

When I was going into the operating room, there was still prepping and everything going on around me. They had my face turned to the side where the operation was going to take place. I also had a thin sheet slightly covering me. I was not able to see much, but I heard a woman's voice come into the room. "Who is this patient?" She asked the surgeon.

"Her name is Valerie Blackwood." He responded. The woman walked over, and I could hear the turning of pages, as she started looking through my medical chart. "What are you preparing to do with this patient?" She asked.

"I am going to take a piece of lymph node out from behind her ear."

"I would also like to have a piece." She requested.

"Yes ma'am." The surgeon agreed. The woman then went on to tell the operating doctors that she wanted me as her patient. With my face still turned, she came over to me. In her soft spoken voice, she politely introduced herself.

"Hello Valerie, my name is Dr. Lawrence. Try not to worry. Everything is going to be fine. I'm going to be handling your case now." She said kindly. I was so relieved by her warm presence.

Medications were given, and I drifted off to sleep. After everything was over and I returned back to my room, my parents were patiently waiting for me. I was so glad to see them. I was feeling so nauseous and began throwing up. I could not even look at the tray of food that was left for me to eat. I was too sick to eat anything at all.

When my test results for the lymph nodes came back, they turned out to be negative. They continued to take many more blood tests and then discharged me on February 18, 1969. I was referred to Jacobi Hospital's Arthritis Clinic on February 26, 1969, where I would be meeting with Dr. Lawrence.

The Diagnosis

On February 26, 1969 at 9:30 AM, I was being seen as a new patient on the third floor of Jacobi Hospital's Arthritis Clinic. I was a little nervous because I did not know what to expect or what Dr. Lawrence was going to say during that visit.

When my name was called, Dr. Lawrence was delighted to see me. As soon as Dr. Lawrence sat down with my mother and I, the first thing that my mother asked was, "Does my daughter have cancer?"

"No, Valerie does not have cancer." Dr. Lawrence replied. My mother was so relieved to hear that. Dr.

Lawrence started looking through my chart. She explained that, when I was in the hospital the last time she saw me, I had taken some blood tests that she was not able to get the results of by the time I was discharged.

Since that time, Dr. Lawrence said that all of my lab results had come back. She said the tests showed that I have what is called Systemic Lupus Erythematosus (SLE). My mother and I were puzzled because it was something we had never heard of before. She told us that there was no cure, but with proper medical treatment, I could continue to live a normal and happy life. Dr. Lawrence started telling us that lupus was a very complicated and unpredictable disease and that it varies from person to person. She said that was why, for so long, I was experiencing rashes on my cheeks, excessive joint pain and swelling, kidney infection, and everything else that I was going through. She said it was all due to the lupus. She told us that lupus could affect any part of the body at any given time.

My mother told Dr. Lawrence, that she knew from the very beginning that everything I had been going through was definitely not Arthritis. Dr. Lawrence agreed and apologized for what I had dealt with. I began taking Prednisone, which is a steroid used to treat numerous medical conditions, and would continue to see Dr. Lawrence at the Arthritis Clinic for my lupus. We had been searching for answers to my health problems for a very long time. I was so relieved that my family and I finally found the answers we were looking for.

Out of School Due to Illness and Was Reinstated

Living with lupus and being constantly sick was not easy for me. I had been out of school and in the hospital for a long while. I had missed so much work in all of my classes. In order for me to be reinstated back in school, my mother had to have all of the necessary forms filled out by the hospital. One of the forms stated that I had Systemic Lupus Erythematosus, that physical activity should not be limited, and that I was under treatment. After all of that was done, I was able to continue on with my eleventh grade classes.

The school advised me that the excused absences did not guarantee a passing mark. They said that my work must be passing. I was so scared. I knew that it was close to the end of the school term and that I would be struggling, but I could not let my lupus get me down. I worked extremely hard and continued to catch up on the work that I had missed. To make a long story short, I did what I had to do and my grades were excellent! I could not believe how well I did. I was able to move on to the twelfth grade. That was such a blessing for me.

Since school was out for the summer, I gave myself a backup plan just in case I got sick during my twelfth grade school year. I decided that I would go to school in the evenings, since I would be working during the day, and double up on some extra classes.

Working for the Neighborhood Youth Corps

During the summer of 1969, I was excited to be working

for The City of New York's Neighborhood Youth Corps as a teacher's aide. It was an exhilarating experience for me. At first, I thought I would not be able to work, but I did not let my health hold me back.

I was taking two medications. I was on 25 mgs of Prednisone per day. Prednisone helped to relieve all of the pain that I was experiencing in my joints. I also had to take one INH pill, to prevent tuberculosis from occurring.

After taking Prednisone on a daily basis, my face started filling out. I felt like I was exploding because of how much Prednisone my doctor had me taking. Working a summer job and feeling my body swell as a reaction to the Prednisone, I could feel that people were taking notice. Everyone could see that something was wrong with me. My face was very round and my weight shot up to about 150 pounds. I was feeling embarrassed about going to work looking the way I did. I told my boss that I was on a lot of medication and that I had to see my doctor on a monthly basis. My boss admitted that he knew something was wrong. He gave me the permission I needed to take time off so that I would be able to see my doctor. He was a wonderful boss and always treated everyone with kindness and respect. I could feel his sincerity and sympathy towards me. He would always praise my work and tell me that I was doing a great job.

After my summer position had ended, I received a Teacher's-Aide Training Program Certificate for the work that I had done. It was issued to me from the Office of Continuing Education, Board of Education, City of New York. I will always treasure this accomplishment.

Getting up early in the morning and walking to work everyday was fantastic motivation for me. It definitely gave me the strength and the physical activity that I really needed to get me through each day. I also attended school in the evenings and felt better about the way things were going for me. My sister, Vanessa, had already taken some of the same classes that I would be taking when I entered twelfth grade so, whenever I needed extra help, she was always there to assist me. I appreciated that so much.

Twelfth Grade

My summer vacation had ended and school was back in session. I prayed that my twelfth grade school year would be much better for me. One morning, when I was quietly sitting in my homeroom class, we heard a knock on our classroom door. My teacher went to open the door, and it was one of the ladies from the main office. She quietly spoke with my teacher. Immediately after, she requested the student's attention, then asked, "Where is Valerie Blackwood?" I instantly became nervous. I did not know what was going on as I cautiously raised my hand.

"Valerie, you have already completed the required commercial course of studies before your scheduled graduation date. Therefore, if you would like to…the school is willing to let you graduate earlier. That means you will not be graduating with your classmates in June as was originally planned. You will now have the opportunity to graduate four months from now, if you would like." She announced.

I was shocked, surprised, and felt incredible inside. I could not believe what was happening to me.

"Would you like to graduate earlier, instead of with your classmates in June?" She asked. "Yes!" I answered gladly and eagerly as I took the opportunity presented to me. She smiled and said that she would head back to the office and make sure that my records were changed accordingly to reflect January, 1970 as my new graduation date. She also said that she would make sure that there was a job lined up for me immediately after graduation. Wow! I could not wait to get out of high school.

My High School Graduation

Graduation time came before I knew it. I was actually not looking forward to attending my own graduation ceremony, but I knew I had to. My face was so fat and my hair was falling out terribly. I wore braided hairpieces just to cover up all of the thinning spots on my head. I was feeling disgusted with myself and just wanted to get that whole evening over with.

My family was really looking forward to the event as they showed their support. They knew how badly I was feeling, but despite all odds, they were happy for what I had accomplished. After my graduation exercises were over, I admittedly felt a little better. It really was a very nice ceremony after all.

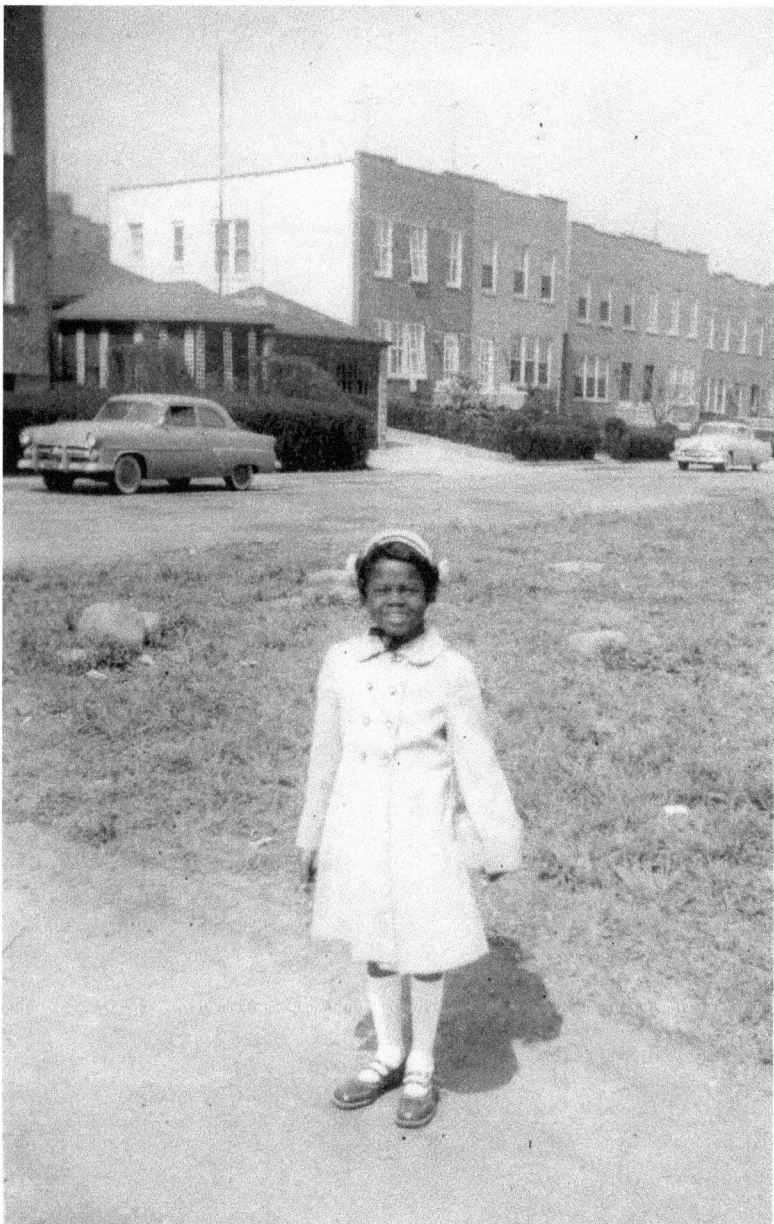

I was five years old and living in Throggs Neck.

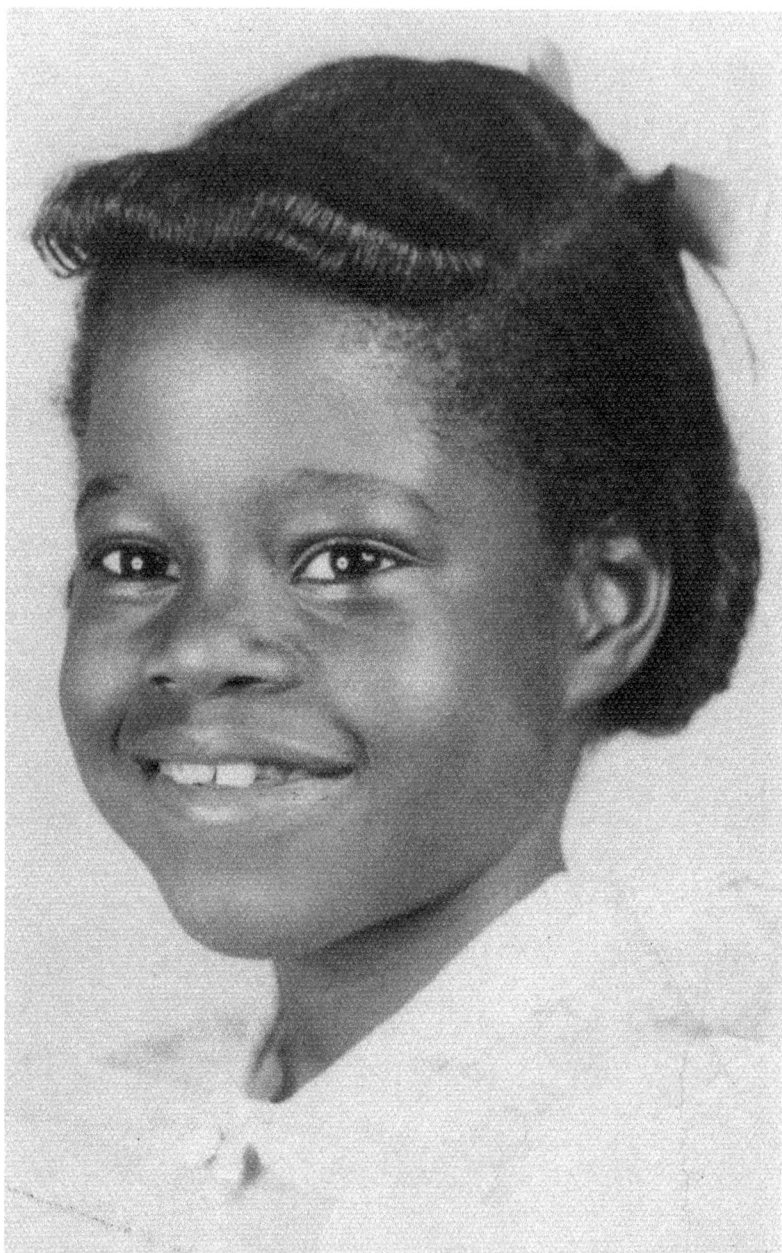

My picture was taken at P.S. 72 in the Bronx. I was six years old.

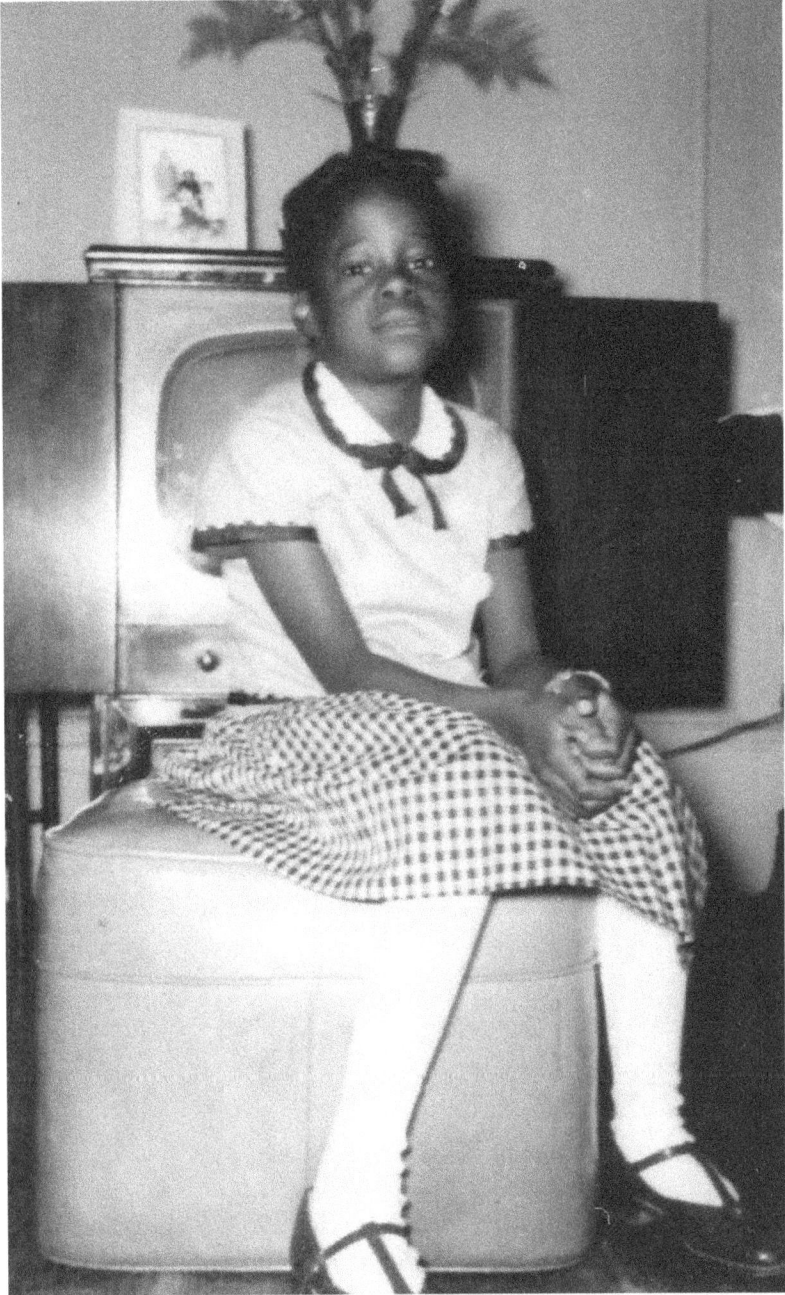

At Uncle Reggie's (my father's brother) house during October 1958.
I was six years old.

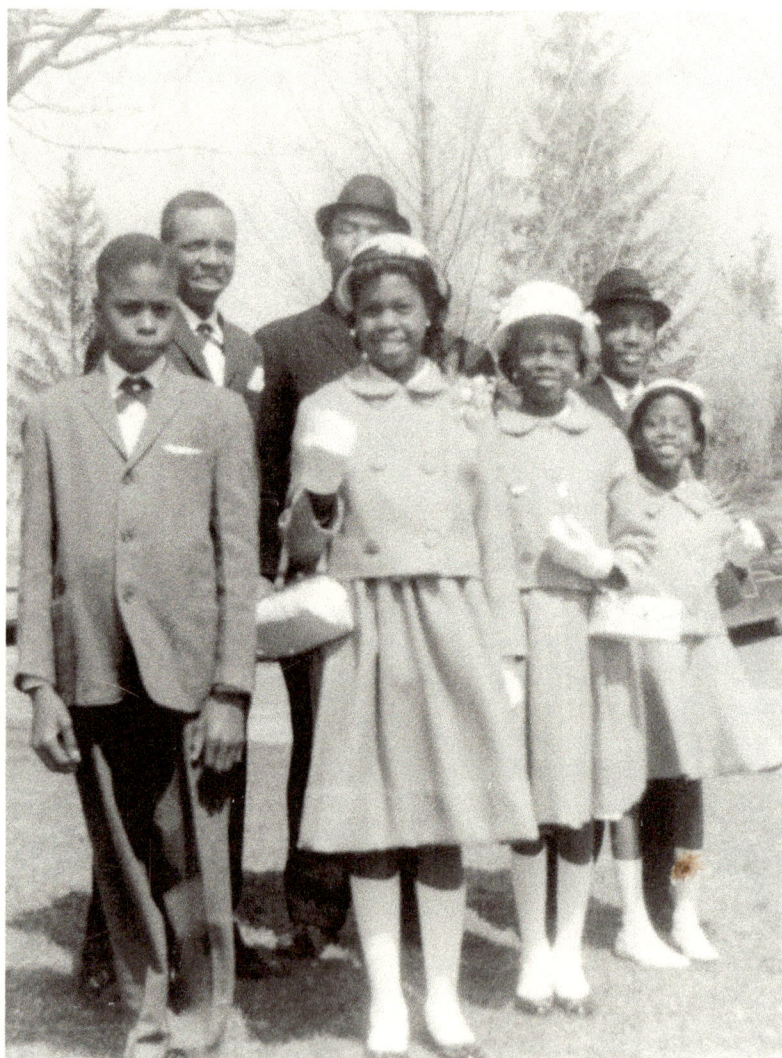

Soon to Become One Big Family

Picture taken by my mother Easter Sunday 1962. Back left to right: Alonzo, Major Colley, Sr., and Junior. Their sister, Etta Mae was not in the picture. Front left to right: My brother, Reginald, sister Vanessa, myself, and my youngest sister, Claudette. (Our mother made the girl's suits).

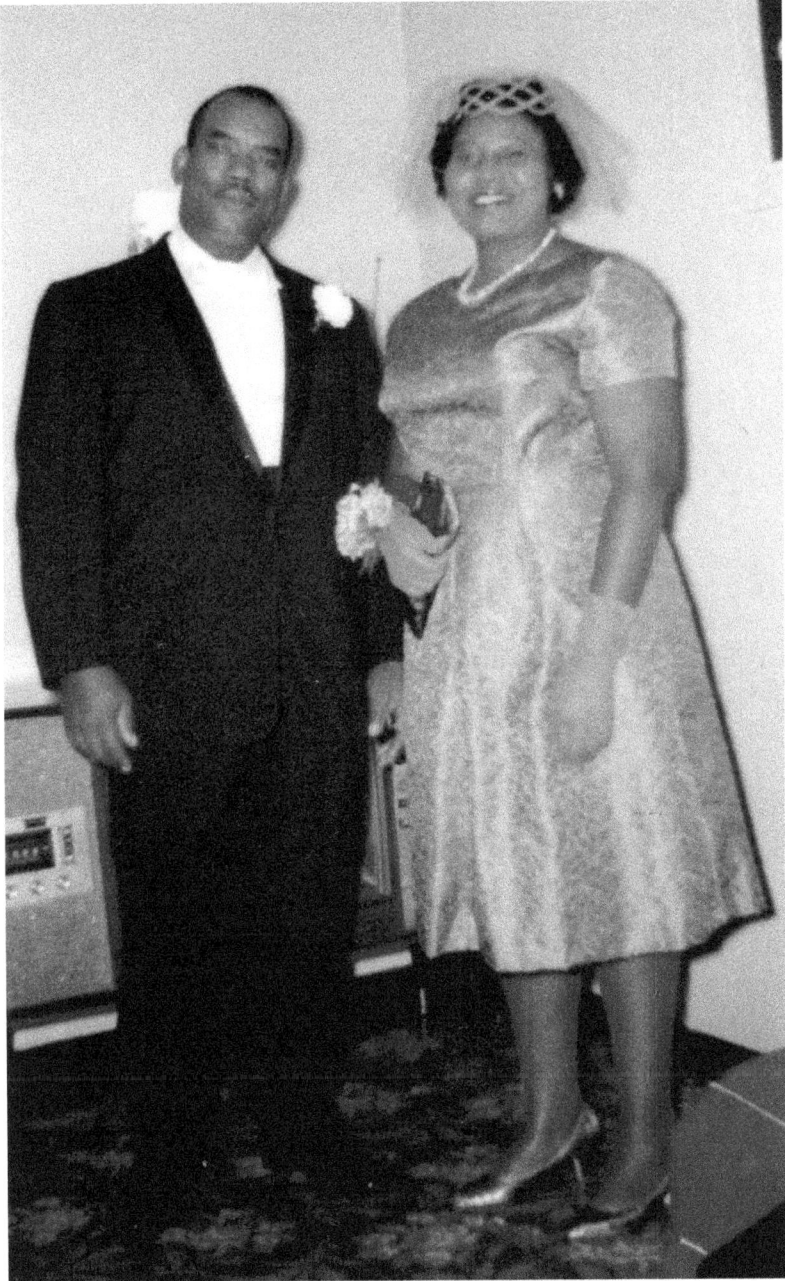

My mother re-married - November 10, 1962
I have a new stepfather, Major Colley, Sr.

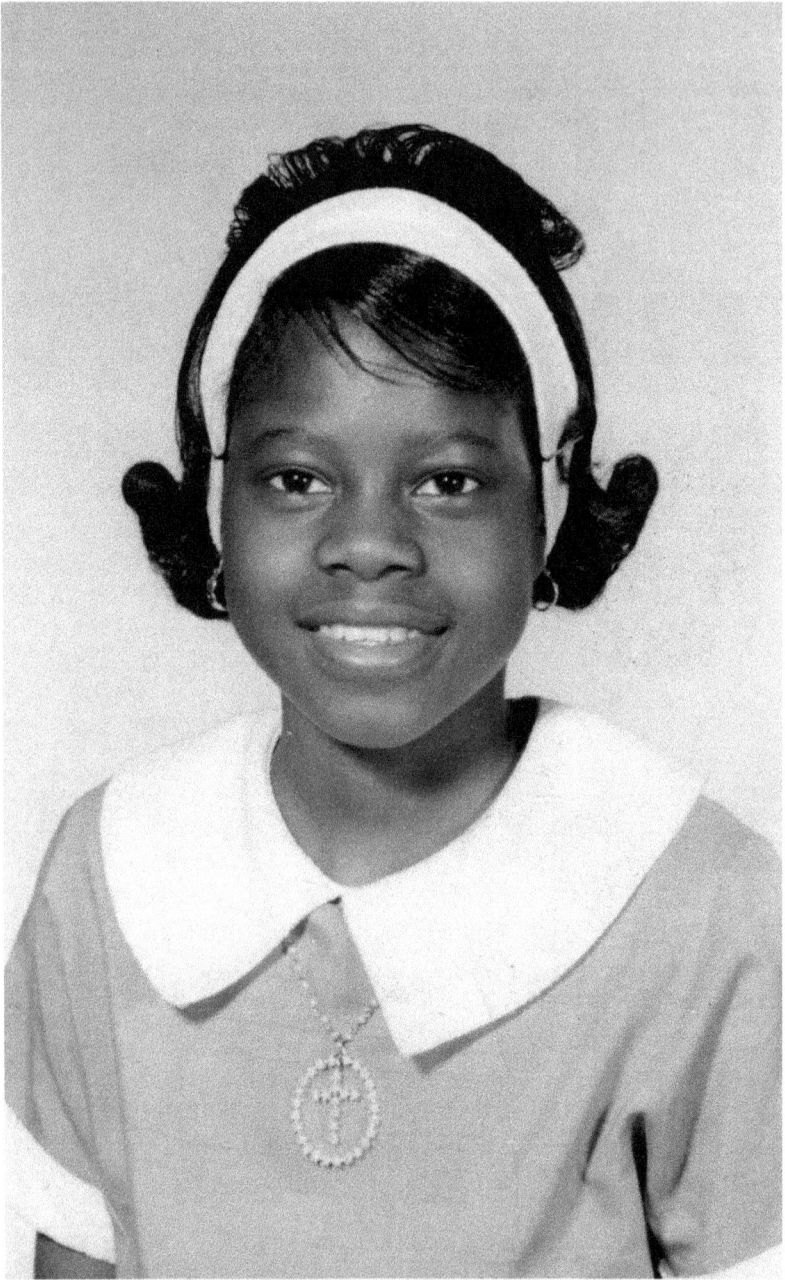

New Neighborhood/New School: Picture taken at school during the springtime of 1964. I was eleven years old.

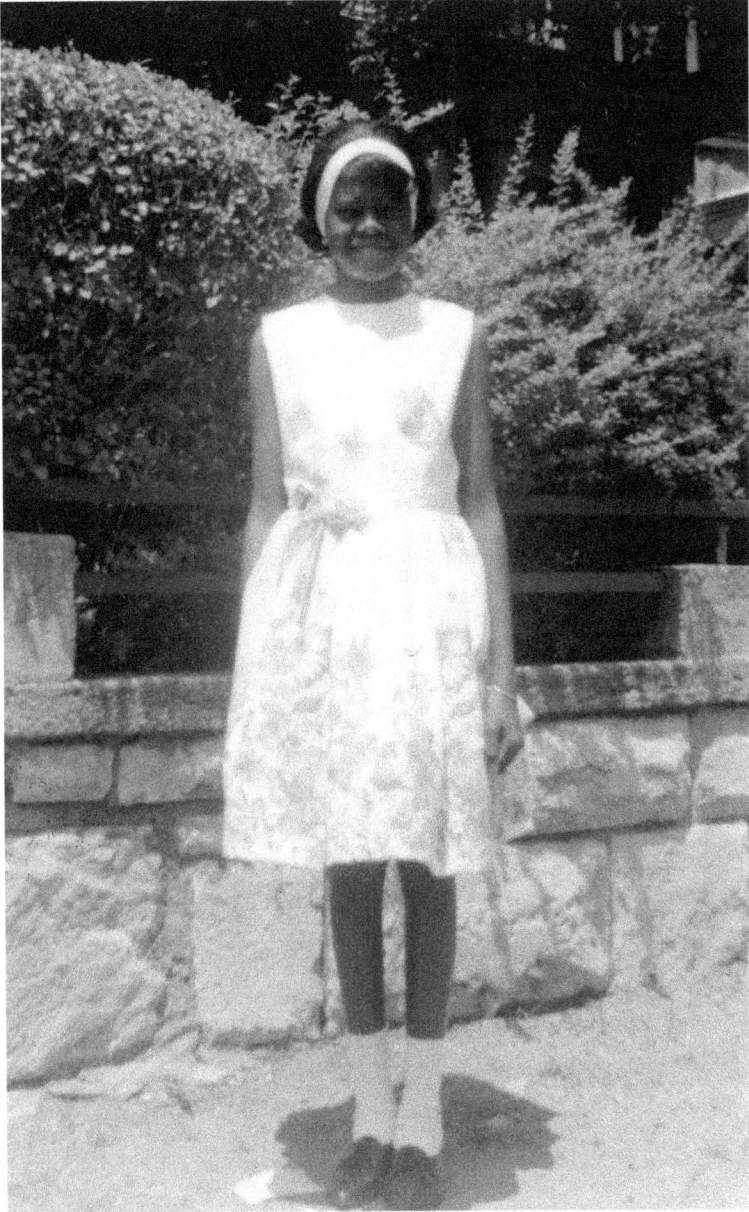

New Neighborhood/New School: Graduating from sixth grade -
Summer of 1964. I was twelve years old, and not happy wearing
those 'bobby socks' on my special day.

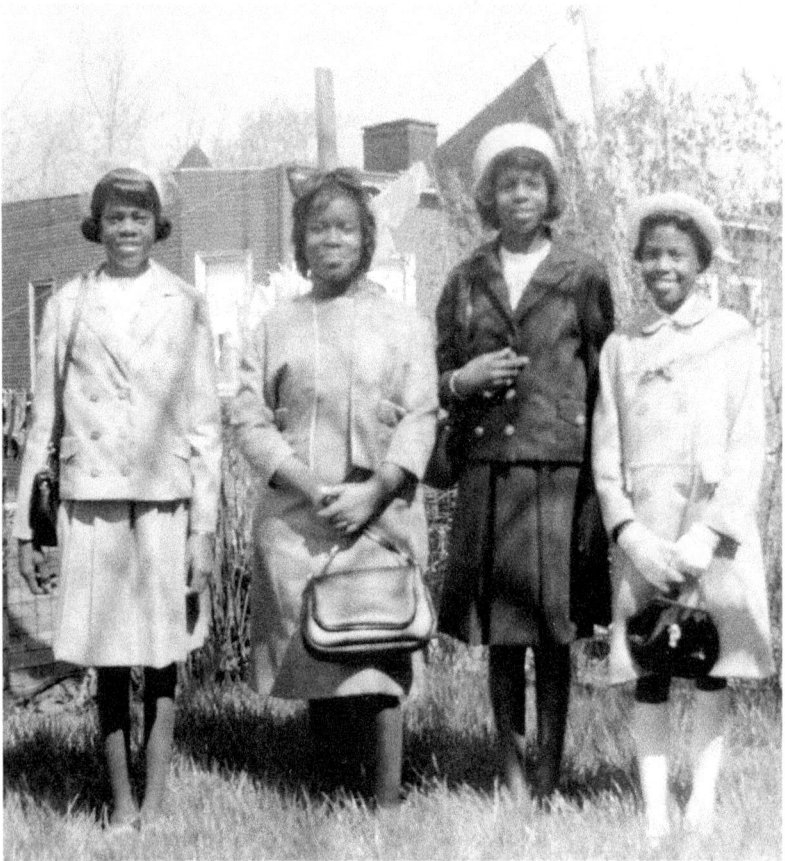

Easter Sunday 1965 in the backyard at our parent's house. Left to right: Me, my stepsister Etta Mae, my sisters Vanessa, and Claudette. (Our mother made our suits).

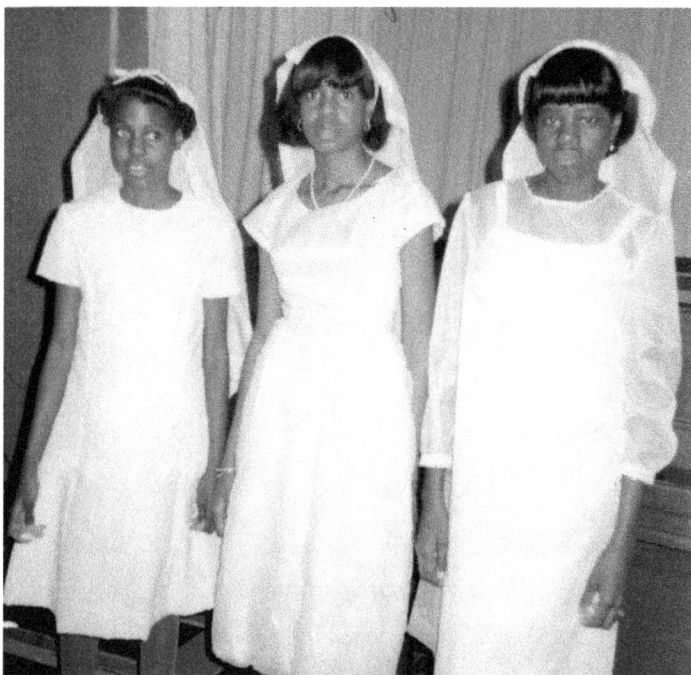

Our Confirmation Day November 27, 1966. (Our mother made our dresses). Left to right: Claudette, Vanessa, and myself.

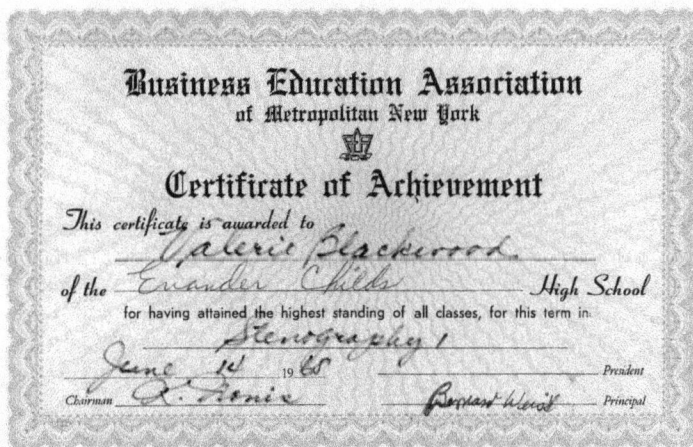

My Big Achievement at Evander Childs High School during June 14, 1968.

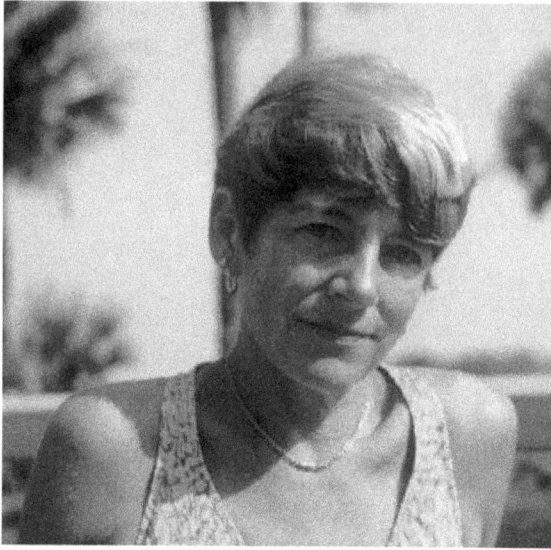

Dr. Christine Lawrence

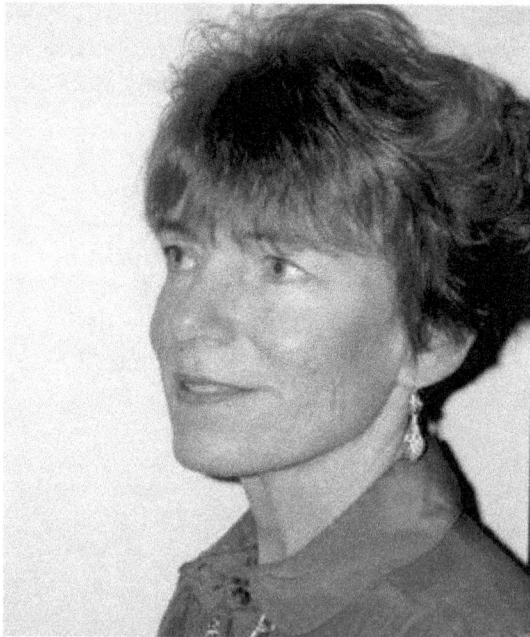

**My lupus diagnosis was received by
Dr. Christine Lawrence.**

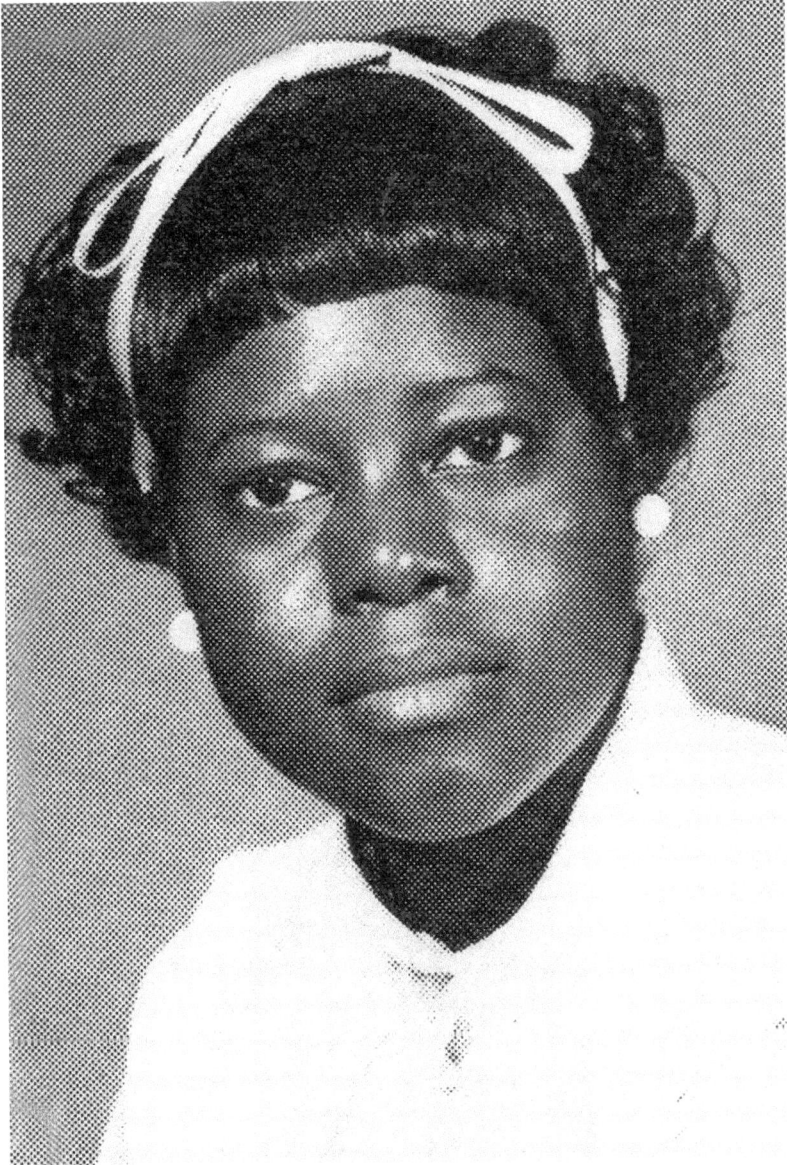

January 1970 graduation yearbook picture - Evander Childs High School. Prednisone medication gave me that round and puffy face.

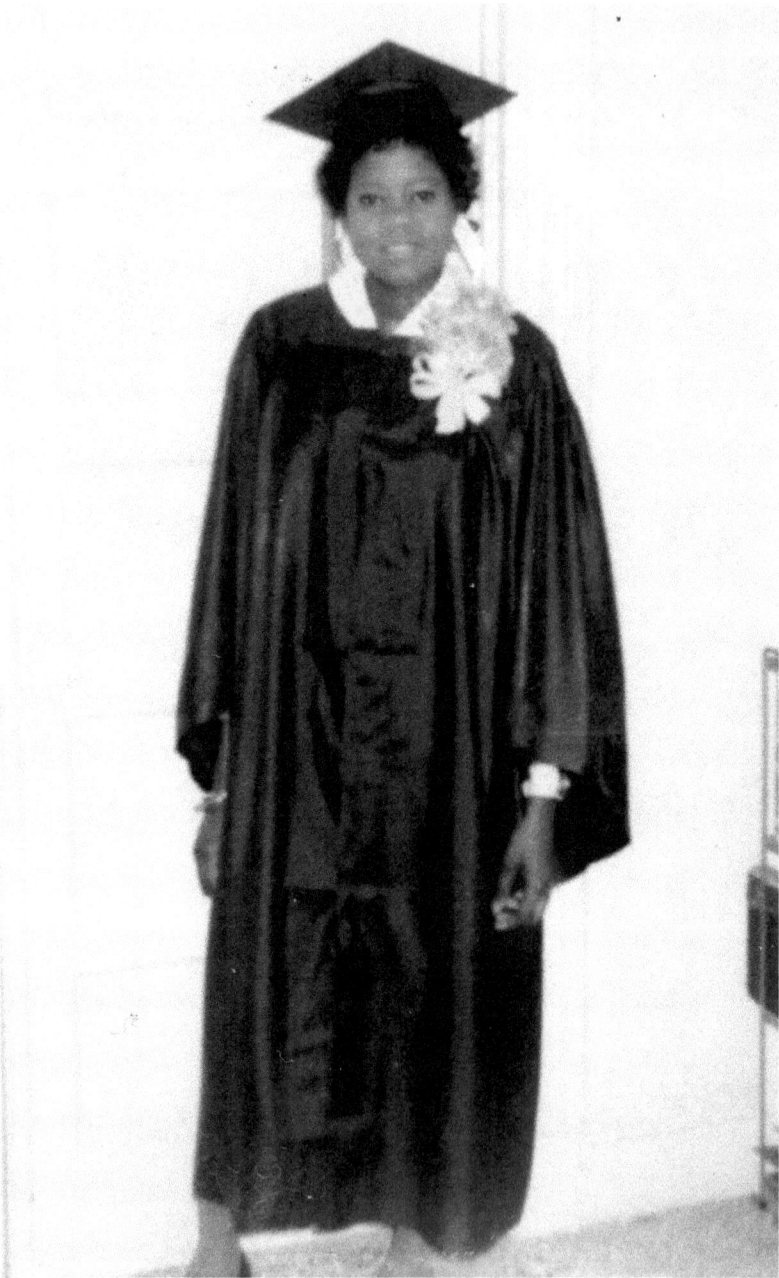

My High School Graduation, January 1970.

CHAPTER 2

LIFE AFTER HIGH SCHOOL

After I graduated from high school, I was still on a very large dose of Prednisone. Dr. Lawrence suggested that I take a new medication called Cytoxin. That pill did not agree with me at all. It was awful, horrible, and made me extremely sick. It gave me stabbing pains in my stomach. It felt as if someone was taking a knife and cutting my stomach wide open. It also caused much of my hair to fall out. After alerting Dr. Lawrence about the side effects I was experiencing, I had to immediately stop taking it. Dr. Lawrence said not to worry, that my hair would definitely grow back. At first, I really didn't believe her, but it did start to grow back slowly.

I had also developed lesions on my face, on the right and left cheek. At first, they were red, and then they turned black. Dr. Lawrence prescribed Kenalog Cream 0.1% and Kenalog Ointment 0.1% for the rashes on my face. I had to start wearing makeup just to cover up the rashes. Then, my breasts started getting all red and felt as if they were on fire. I could not put anything on them to relieve the discomfort. I would just wash gently with a mild soap and water. My legs, thighs, and buttocks were all scarred with stretch marks from being on so much Prednisone. The marks were so deep that I could put my fingers inside each crevice of my skin. Dr. Lawrence said that in due time they would slowly go away.

Working at the Bank

At the age of seventeen and a half, I started working at the bank as a junior secretary to the vice president. That was the job my school referred me to once I graduated. My sister, Vanessa, was also working there, but in a different department. After working there for just a short period of time, the atmosphere did not feel good to me at all. My boss always kept a stern look on his face and was not at all pleasant to work with. I knew that he definitely did not want this young, black girl, straight out of high school to be working for him, but I was assigned to that position and had the skills necessary.

One day, my boss approached me while I was sitting at my desk. He told me that I needed to see Personnel. So, I immediately went to their office. I could not believe it! My boss had the nerve to ask Personnel to issue me another secretarial test to take. I took the test and passed it. I knew that my nerves had gotten the best of me and that I would not be able to do the job that I was assigned. I could not work there under those conditions. Therefore, I told my sister how I was feeling and decided that the best thing for me to do was to leave. I was so relieved to be out of there and I started looking for another job as fast as I could.

Around the same time that I had left my job, I also had an appointment at Jacobi Hospital's Arthritis Clinic. I was so happy that my health was not affected by my work. I was feeling pretty good, and I kept taking my Prednisone pills as instructed.

Working for the Boys' Clubs of America

During May of 1970, we had such beautiful weather in New York City. After I received a referral from the New York State Unemployment Office in the Bronx, I started working for the Boys' Clubs of America as a secretary in the Human Resources Department. I also would help out at the switchboard. I enjoyed my new position and really appreciated working there. Everyone was so nice and easy to get along with. I also received the okay from my superior that I be given a few hours off each month in order to see my doctor. The end of 1970 turned out to be a memorable year for me because I had a great job that I really loved.

We had beautiful weather during May, 1971. I could not believe how fast the time had gone. I had already been working at the Boys' Clubs of America for one year. I was feeling the stability of my job: I felt more energetic, and looked forward to going out and having fun. I was almost nineteen years old when I started dating.

One Saturday night, my cousin, Verona, and I went out to a club. I met someone interesting and we exchanged telephone numbers by the end of the evening. His name was Ben. Ben called me that following day. When I was speaking with him on the telephone, I found out that he was a twin. I could hear his twin brother, Robert, in the background saying to him, "You know you are seeing someone else and going back home next week." Ben responded to his brother by hushing him, "Be quiet." His twin said to him, "Why don't you let me talk to her." So, he gave Robert the telephone and we spoke. He told me that Ben spoke so highly of me after we met at the club. After speaking to Robert, I felt a genuine connection with him and the conversation did not feel forced at all. We decided that, since his brother was just visiting and ready to go back to Alabama, we would meet each other at the same club that following Saturday.

When I met Robert, they sounded just alike, but I was able to tell them apart. They were fraternal twins. He was slightly taller than his brother and seemed very nice. He was dark skinned, over six feet tall, and had a slender build. His age was also perfect for me; there was not even a full year age difference between us. He was born and raised in Alabama and decided to live in New York City. Being with him made me so happy. We got along so well and immediately started dating. I was still on Prednisone pills and my round face was showing like a moon, but I always made sure to take my Prednisone pills at the same time each day.

On June 2, 1971 I started having problems with my feet. They were constantly swelling and felt very hot to the touch, but I was not experiencing any pain at all. Since my birthday was coming that month, I was hoping that my health would improve.

My period did not come at all during the months of May, June, and July 1971. When the month of August came, I was feeling strong and my period finally came. I did not have a heavy flow at all and I did not experience any pain or discomfort. It felt like it wasn't even there and only lasted about five days. From September 1971 all the way into December, my period still had not come.

On December 31, 1971, my parents were hosting a party at their house. My mother and father were busy getting so many things ready for the evening. As we were setting up the décor in the dining room—it was so funny—my youngest sister, Claudette, my mother, and my grandmother decided to try out their individual horns for the party. I wanted to take a picture of them doing that; it was definitely a moment worth capturing. As the evening went on, our family and friends were there to celebrate that festive night as we brought in the New Year. My boyfriend had a great time being with my family. I enjoyed being with him every month, even though we usually only saw each other on the weekends. After knowing Robert for just that period of time, we already knew that we would be together and one day get married. So, we started saving our money.

On February 9, 1972, I started working in another position at the Boys' Clubs of America. I was chosen to work as a secretary to the assistant of the company. I was continuously seeing Dr. Lawrence at the Arthritis Clinic at Jacobi Hospital. I was taking two and a half 5 mg Prednisone pills daily, plus two INH pills daily. At night, I would also take Maalox tablets to give my stomach a coating.

Oftentimes, I felt like just sitting around and doing absolutely nothing. I just didn't have the energy, it seemed. I kept getting hot flashes and I was only nineteen years old. I did not know what was going on. I could not believe that I would have to wake up in the middle of the night and change from winter pajamas back into summer pajamas. I was sweating like mad. I would take off my socks only to put them back on, again and again. That seemed like all I ever did. I also started to notice that my heart would race if I worked just a little too hard.

On March 8, 1972, I had a clinic appointment. It was an extremely rainy day outside in New York City. I noticed that the skin on the top part of my right hand had turned black and blue. My hand felt hot to the touch and a little sore. Dr. Lawrence suggested that I start taking my Prednisone pills this way: On Monday, Wednesday, and Friday, I should take two 5 mg Prednisone pills, and on all the other days, I should take two and a half 5 mg Prednisone pills. Dr. Lawrence was trying to slowly reduce the amount of pills I was taking.

I was still loving my job and happy to be working there. After having another clinic appointment with Dr. Lawrence, she said my health was improving. After months of not having my period, it finally came on May 15, 1972—which was a long time for me. I was advised to start taking two 5 mg Prednisone pills daily, two INH pills daily, and later at night, two Maalox No. 2 tablets. I did not experience any aches or pains and my weight leveled at 134 pounds. Dr. Lawrence was able to reduce my Prednisone just a little.

When my birthday came in June, I turned twenty years old. I did not get my period that month; I also did not have any hot flashes. When I saw Dr. Lawrence, she said that things seemed to be going very well for me. I could really see things improving. During my clinic appointment, I was still taking two 5 mg Prednisone pills and two INH pills. At that time, Dr. Lawrence did not want anything to change just yet. She wanted to get my urine and blood test results before deciding exactly what she wanted to do.

Normally, I would see Dr. Lawrence on a monthly basis, but she had me skip the month of August 1972. That was a test to see how my health would hold up without seeing her for evaluation. I did not mind at all. It was good for me because I did not have to miss any extra time away from work.

I had a clinic appointment with Dr. Lawrence on September 20th. Dr. Lawrence informed me that everything was okay and that she would see me the following month.

On October 25, 1972, I had a clinic appointment with Dr. Lawrence. She informed me that all of my laboratory tests, such as blood and urine, all seemed fine. She was so pleased, that she reduced my Prednisone pills on every third day, taking one and a half pills. That meant that I would have to take one pill and break the other 5 mg pill in half. For example, starting on October 26th, I would take two Prednisone pills. On the second day I would take two 5 mg Prednisone pills, and on the third day I would take one and a half Prednisone pills, plus my INH pills, and I would keep repeating that method until she told me otherwise.

During the month of November, I did not see my doctor and therefore didn't have to miss any time away from my job. I was still taking my Prednisone pills the same way: (two, two, and one and a half), plus my INH pills.

I was at the clinic the morning of December 6, 1972. I was only there to give a urine sample, but they also took three tubes of blood from me. My doctor would not be reducing my Prednisone dosage until she saw me the following week.

On December 13, 1972 I had an appointment with Dr. Lawrence. My test results appeared to be very good. I was losing weight little by little. My appetite was not at all like it used to be. Dr. Lawrence had another young doctor look at my hands during the visit. She was explaining to him the difference between lupus patients and arthritis patients. She explained to the doctor that if I were not taking any Prednisone pills, my skin would not be as smooth as it should be–it would just draw-up the very same way that the people with arthritis experience, which presents as deformity in their knuckles and fingers. Dr. Lawrence was very proud of the way things had been progressing for me. It was because of this that she did not want to change the way I was taking the Prednisone. She wanted to reduce the pills gradually. She said that if I went too fast, everything would just flare-up again and I would have to start all over by taking larger doses like before—she advised that it was not worth the risk.

When Robert would come to my parent's house to see me, he was always so amazed to see how well our house was kept and how well my mother could sew. Thanks to my mother, those same qualities were instilled in me. Robert knew that I was able to sew, so he bought me a very nice sewing machine with the table attached. On Sundays, my father would read the bible. If there were any friends or family members at the house, he was always ready to share his spiritual knowledge. My father loved having company and he could sit for hours talking.

During the holidays, my siblings and all of our significant others, would be celebrating at my parent's house. My mother's birthday is December 22nd, and my father's birthday is on Christmas Day. The family always had a beautiful time together.

Another new year came around so fast. On January 1, 1973, Dr. Lawrence wanted me to do something a little different because I would not be seeing her for a little while. She wanted me to reverse my Prednisone pills. Her orders were to take: one and a half Prednisone pills on day one, one and a half Prednisone pills on day two, and then two Prednisone pills on day three. I was taking half a pill less than what I was taking before. I only came to the clinic to give a urine sample and have my blood drawn on January 31, 1973. Dr. Lawrence told me that, if anything should develop before then, I should see her immediately.

From February 1973 through April 1973, my health was stabilizing and nothing serious had developed. At that time, I was taking one and a half Prednisone pills daily. Dr. Lawrence told me that she would be going on vacation in May, so I would not see her during that time. She continued to tell me how well I was doing and that she was very proud of me. Plus, my blood tests also looked good.

During the month of May, I had an open conversation with Robert about lupus and how it has affected me. After speaking with him, I was very surprised that he took it so calmly. He said, "My baby is just sick." He also mentioned that he hoped it wouldn't affect my ability to have children. I planned on speaking with my doctor about that at our next appointment.

On Wednesday, June 6, 1973, I had a clinic appointment. Dr. Lawrence was steadily keeping me down to one and a half Prednisone pills daily. My health was steady, but I was experiencing a little swelling around the ankles every now and then. When I sat down with Dr. Lawrence, I had one question that I needed to ask her.

"Can I have children?" I asked her.

"I see no reason why you having lupus should stop you from having children." She replied. I was so relieved to hear her say that—especially because years prior, she and the other doctors had told me that I probably would not be able to have a child. She also commented on how things were moving along so nicely for me. After seeing Dr. Lawrence, I was eating much less. I did not have a very good appetite. It was hard to eat a decent breakfast in the morning. When I would try to eat, I would take just a few little bites and throw the rest of the food away because it made me feel so nauseous.

During the latter part of June, I surprised Robert with a dashiki shirt that I made for him from the very nice sewing machine he purchased for me. He wore the shirt when we went to the Bronx Zoo that summer.

We experienced extremely hot weather in New York

City in July 1973. After I turned twenty-one, I experienced some ups and downs in my health. I had to stop using the prescribed Kenalog Cream at 0.1% that Dr. Lawrence had prescribed for my skin. It made my face too dry. Dr. Lawrence informed me that they had discontinued the Kenalog Ointment at 0.1% that I always used. I was not happy to hear that and was hoping to get more. That Kenalog Ointment was excellent when I used it. I never experienced any pimples or bumps on my face. It made my skin very moist.

When the month of July was almost over, my face started breaking out with small pimples. They looked like small blisters that turned red and then black. It itched terribly. I tried my best not to scratch. The only thing that I was putting on my face was a little Vaseline. I would put it on once in the morning and at nighttime. I did not know if it was helping me at all. Also, my eating habits seemed to be somewhat off-balanced because I did not have the taste for any breakfast at all. I ate fairly well at dinner and was able to sleep good at night. My weight did not increase or decrease – it pretty much stayed the same. I was also moving my bowels so often that it seemed like my insides were coming out of me. My feet would still swell at night, but I did not have any pain.

I was so glad that the pimples and blisters breaking out on my face were slowly starting to show improvement and eventually they cleared up altogether. When I had my clinic appointment with Dr. Lawrence, she told me that I should not use any Vaseline on my face because it would only clog my pores. My eating habits were normal and my weight was ideal at 123 pounds.

On December 12, 1973, I had a clinic appointment with Dr. Lawrence. The first thing that Dr. Lawrence told me was how nicely I was doing and that everything was looking good. She advised me that on Tuesdays and Fridays, I would start taking one and a half 5 mg Prednisone pills and on the other days, I would take only one 5 mg Prednisone pill. I also had some lab work done. Dr. Lawrence told me to please call her back on December 19, 1973 to get the results of the blood work.

I was unable to call Dr. Lawrence at that time. Therefore, my mother spoke with her. She informed my mother that everything looked very good and that I should now only take one 5 mg Prednisone pill each day. I was really happy to hear that. When I started on that small dose, I still was feeling very good. The only change that I noticed was that I was getting little sores inside my ears. They became very dry and scaly. I would sometimes scratch because my ears itched so badly. I put a little Vaseline inside, just to keep it moist.

My parents had a very nice New Year's Eve party that year. My father always looked forward to entertaining. He was also a great cook. Our family and friends were there to celebrate. New Year's Eve turned out to be beautiful.

On January 30, 1974 I had an appointment to see Dr. Lawrence. During that visit she said that everything was continuing to improve. So, she decided to give me a four-month long test without seeing her at the clinic. I was so glad that I would not have to come so often.

We were supposed to be taking our honeymoon to Robert's hometown in Alabama, but his mother had passed away on April 24th. That was such a horrific time in Robert's life and it took a real toll on him. We decided that we would not be taking a honeymoon.

Since I was already engaged, my Aunt Muriel asked me, "Valerie, have you tested the waters yet?" I told her, "No." She encouraged me to find out if he was actually a He/He or a He/She. I felt that it made sense, so we did it...just once. I felt so embarrassed because, after withholding from sex for all of those years, Robert's condom was forgotten in the toilet and my mother found it while she was having company. After that happened, I said I was going to wait until marriage. Robert and I started apartment hunting. We were able to find a very nice apartment in a three family house. Robert would be living there until we got married.

New York City's weather was beautiful during May 1, 1974. That was the next time that Dr. Lawrence saw me since my four-month long break. She was so proud that I was doing so well. "Valerie, you are one of my best patients because you do everything just right." She told me. That was so nice of her to say. I looked at her, smiled, and said, "Thank you." My weight was 118¾ pounds. I couldn't believe how much my weight had come down. There were no more weighted down pounds from all of the Prednisone I was taking. It felt great! During that visit, Dr. Lawrence instructed me on how to alter my Prednisone medication. She said that on Mondays, I should take half of a 5 mg Prednisone pill. The other days, I should take one 5 mg Prednisone pill. That was probably one of the best visits I had with my doctor.

On May 17, 1974, Robert and I started looking for

bedroom furniture. We were able to find a very nice set that we both liked. Things were going good for us. On June 8, our bedroom set was delivered to our new apartment and Robert was able to move in. At least we no longer had to worry about where we were going to live.

Less than two weeks before our wedding, Robert showed me a side of himself that I had never ever seen before. He would get so angry when we discussed things that needed to be finalized before the wedding. I could not understand why he was getting so angry. I told him to calm down because these were things that we needed to take care of before our wedding day. I did not like that side of him at all, let alone right before our wedding.

I told my mother that I was having some doubts about getting married. Her response to me was, "If you don't know what to do, Valerie, just stand still and don't do anything." My mother and father had done so much for us already and it was just a week before my wedding—I just could not bring myself to do that.

I was thinking back to what my father had said to me when he first met Robert. He told me that he was a hardworking, southern young man and that was one of the qualities you must look for in a man. When I told my grandmother (my mother's mother) what my father had said, her response to me was, "He is saying that because he is also a southern man who is very hardworking, but you have to do what you think is best for yourself."

As I thought about everything up until now, I put all of those feelings aside. I knew, without a doubt in my mind, that I truly loved Robert and that he was truly in love with me; I looked forward to getting married.

On Wednesday, July 10, 1974, just a few days before my wedding, I had an appointment to see Dr. Lawrence. After seeing her, she told me that everything looked good and that she expected that I would continue doing well.

On July 12th, my siblings, aunts and uncles were at my parent's house. Everyone was helping with last minute preparations for tomorrow's big day. My mother had made my wedding dress, my maid of honor's dress, and my girlfriend's dress, but my cousin, Pat had her dress made by her sister, Anita. Later that evening, I was helping my mother put lovely beads on my dress. It was a beautiful moment that I got to share with her.

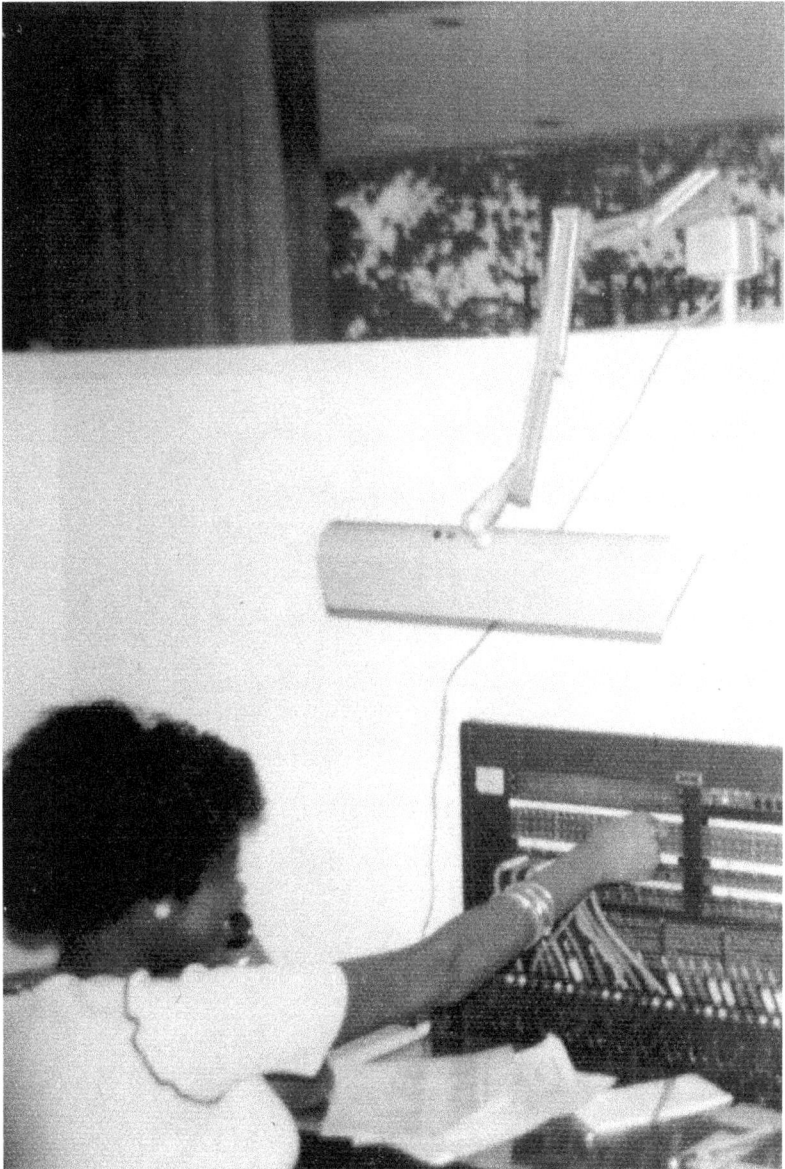

*I was a secretary, as well as a relief switchboard operator
at Boys' Clubs of America – May 1970.*

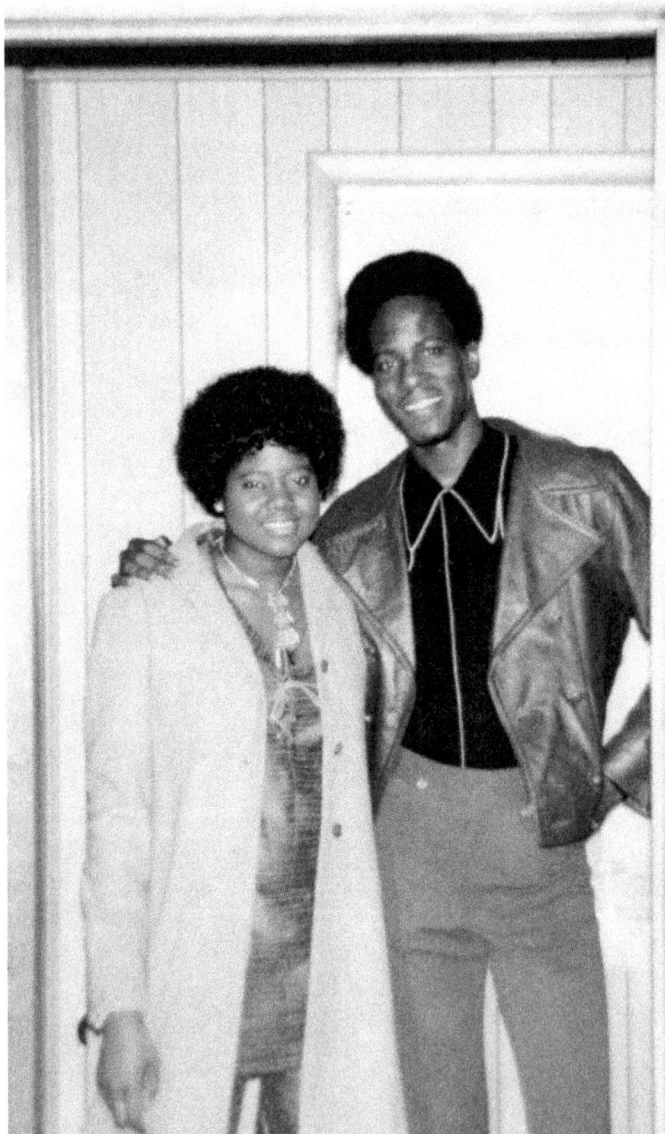

Robert and I were on our way to a Club.
Prednisone medication gave me that round and puffy face.

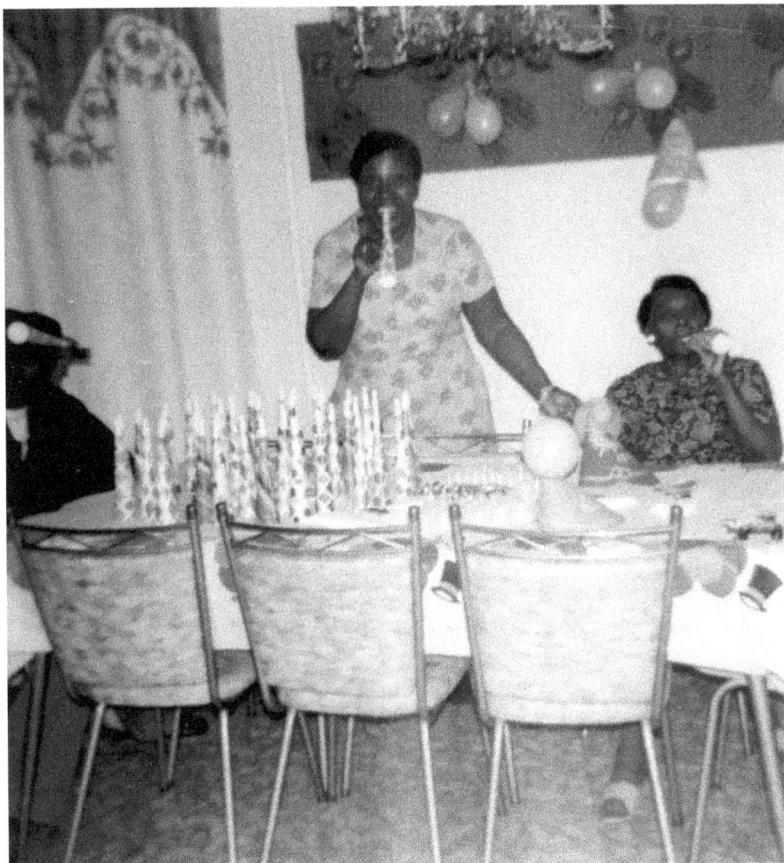

Our parents were hosting a New Year's Eve Party. Left to right: My sister, Claudette, my mother, and grandmother were trying out their horns.

CHAPTER 3

MARRIED LIFE

Saturday, July 13, 1974 was my big day. It was my Wedding Day! My wedding ceremony took place at St. Luke's Episcopal Church in the Bronx, New York. The reception immediately following, took place in my parent's backyard. As the evening went on, I changed into a long, red halter dress. Our family and friends were there to celebrate that most wonderful occasion! There was so much food and drinks that it lasted all the way into the wee hours of the night. My wedding turned out beautifully. I was the last one out of my seven siblings living at home to get married. But, my mother and father still had my grandmother (my mother's mother) and their two foster children Lisa and Barry at home. So, their house was not going to be lonely.

Since Robert and I were not going on a honeymoon, we stayed over at my parent's house because we had so many beautiful gifts to bring to our apartment. After a couple of days flew by, Robert was not making a move to leave my parent's house. He was getting a little too comfortable there. My mother even asked me, "When is he planning on leaving? You have a very nice apartment, it's time for both of you to be in your own place." I realized that married life had hit him and he was scared. Our life together had officially begun.

On October 16, 1974, I met with Dr. Lawrence. She said that things were still going really well for me. She decided to decrease my Prednisone pills to a half a pill on Mondays, Wednesdays, and Fridays, and on the other days, I would only take one Prednisone pill. As the year of 1974 came to a close, I did not have to see my doctor.

On January 8, 1975, I went to Jacobi Hospital just to have my blood drawn. At 8:00 PM, I went to my parent's house. I had a very bad nosebleed, which lasted about thirty minutes.

I also had significant blood clots, which almost choked me to death. When the bleeding finally stopped, I went home. After returning back home, I started washing my face and my nose began bleeding all over again. It was so bad that I had to put some vinegar on a piece of tissue and put it in my nose. Robert called the police and they referred us to the nearest hospital. They also told us to put some ice on the nose. It helped a little, but it still continued to bleed. So, around 10:00 PM that night, we took a taxi to Jacobi Hospital. When we arrived, the hospital took a little blood from my finger. They also checked my blood pressure and my pulse and everything appeared to be okay. After the bleeding subsided, the hospital did not want to do anything further since I had my own doctor at Jacobi Hospital who knew my medical history. After we returned back home, everything was much better. Two days later, the hospital called to find out how I was doing. I also had a clinic appointment with Dr. Lawrence on the 15th. She said that my blood tests looked beautiful, but couldn't give an explanation for my bloody nose. I was feeling strong on the day of my clinic visit. She also told me that on Mondays, Wednesdays, Fridays, and Saturdays I should only take a half of a 5 mg Prednisone pill, and on Tuesdays, Thursdays, and Sundays I should take one 5 mg Prednisone pill.

Could I Be Pregnant?

I had been feeling a little funny inside. It was not a good feeling I was having. I thought to myself, "Could I be pregnant?" I felt that if I did become pregnant, I would not be able to stay pregnant for long. That was just the way my body felt to me at the time.

On February 18, 1975, Robert and I rushed to Jacobi Hospital. At that very moment, I was in so much pain. It felt as if all of my insides wanted to come out. I felt like I had to move my bowels, but I just couldn't. I could not even urinate without it causing pain. While sitting in the chair at the hospital, Robert and I waited from 3:00 AM to 8:30 AM for someone to help us. Before leaving that hospital, I rushed to the bathroom and noticed that I had been bleeding. At that point, I was so scared that we immediately took a taxi to Misericordia Hospital. When Robert and I arrived, they immediately gave me a pregnancy test. The test results showed that I was pregnant. I was admitted into the hospital due to the severe pain and bleeding. They started an intravenous in my arm and it seemed to help the pain, but the bleeding continued. The hospital told me that I had an Ectopic pregnancy and was aborting. I could not believe that was happening to me.

I asked the hospital, "How long will all of this take?" I could not believe the response the hospital gave me. They said, "This is a Catholic hospital. We do not do any type of abortions. Therefore, if you stay in this hospital, you will have to abort on your own. We will just watch and make sure that you are as comfortable as possible until it happens." I was so angry that I just wanted to get up and leave because I was in so much pain. I was in no shape to do all that. I just had to wait it out and see what my body was going to do.

When my mother came to visit me in the hospital, I told her that I had to go to the bathroom really bad. When I went to the bathroom, a very long clot of blood came out of me and plopped right into the toilet. I called out to my mother and I told the doctors. They said that was what they were waiting for.

After that happened, I had an EUA (examination under anesthesia) and a D and C (dilation and curettage procedure) on March 4, 1975. The doctor who did the procedure told me that it should also help to regulate my periods. He said, "Within five months you should be able to try to get pregnant again." The doctor did an excellent job. I was so glad that everything was finally over with. I was discharged from the hospital on March 6, 1975.

The doctor was right. After having the D and C, my

period came on time, which was April 2, 1975 and it was a normal flow. It came again on May 1st and again on May 30th.

Explaining to Dr. Lawrence What Happened

When I went to see Dr. Lawrence on June 4, 1975, I told her everything that happened to me, while I was waiting to be seen at Jacobi Hospital. Dr. Lawrence was so angry that she wanted to know the names of the individuals who were on staff that morning when all of that happened. I told her that I was in so much pain I could not even think straight. I told her that all I wanted was for someone to help me and no one ever did. She wanted me to pursue that further because she said I could have died right there. I told her that after so many hours had passed, we finally just got up and went to another hospital. Dr. Lawrence was still extremely angry. When my birthday came that month, I turned twenty-three years old.

One day, during the summer of 1975, my father took the family out to look at some beautiful homes located in Long Island. We were amazed by all the land and the brand new homes we saw. My father always encouraged us to own real estate. I was so mad because Robert completely lacked interest and had no desire to look at anything. He said that he was still young and just not ready for any of that. I was very much interested and went without him. I felt that I would enjoy having my own home one day, especially since we were already renting an apartment in a three family house.

I had a clinic appointment with Dr. Lawrence on July

30, 1975. Dr. Lawrence said that everything was doing fine.

Around September, I was feeling dissatisfied with my married life. I was under a significant amount of stress and feeling very emotional. My period came on September 1st and was over in three days. Then it came back on September 7th and lasted one day. I saw Dr. Lawrence again on September 24th. My period came on October 1, 1975 and again on October 27th. After that my periods were regulated.

My Secretarial Position Was Being Phased Out

I had been working for the Boys' Clubs of America for five and a half years when they informed me that, because of a very tight economy, they found it imperative to go into a contingency budget—which forced them to make considerable cuts in basic expenditures. As a result, the position that was held by my supervisor was being phased out, along with my secretarial position.

I was sorry to see my position with the Boys' Clubs of America end after being there for such a good amount of time. We all knew, previously, that there was going to be some company changes and/or cuts within the departments, but we just didn't know when. All-in-all, I really enjoyed working for the Boys' Clubs of America. That was the beginning of my young adult life, and I learned so much from being with such a great company.

On November 5, 1975, I had a clinic appointment with Dr. Lawrence. After meeting with her, she said that everything was normal and that my lupus was under control. My last day of employment with the Boys' Clubs was on November 14th.

On January 21, 1976, I had an appointment with Dr. Lawrence. Dr. Lawrence decided that on all days except Tuesday, I should take half of a 5 mg Prednisone pill. On Tuesdays, I should only take one 5 mg Prednisone pill.

Dr. Lawrence had been watching my blood results very carefully. She said that it seemed to be a little on the shaky side. Therefore, she had to start me on Ferrous Sulfate, a 325 mg iron pill that had to be taken twice a day. After sitting down with Dr. Lawrence, she asked me, "Valerie, when are you going to have a baby?" She knew what I had gone through the previous February. I told her that I was a little scared. She told me that taking half of a 5 mg Prednisone pill each day would not do any damage to me or a baby. I was very glad to hear her say that, even though that was not on my mind.

When my period came on February 6, 1976, I started to feel quite a bit of discomfort on my left side. I was getting sharp pains that would come and go, and I started to get worried. I thought to myself, *It feels a little like what I was going through when I had my miscarriage.* I realized that it was just a lot of cramping that I was experiencing from my period and then the pain finally went away.

Working With the Juvenile Diabetes Foundation

On March 29, 1976, I started a new position with the Juvenile Diabetes Foundation. I was hired to work as a secretary to the Foundation. I was happy to be working there and I learned so much about diabetes.

June 16, 1976, I had a clinic appointment to see Dr. Lawrence. After meeting with her, she said that everything was doing alright thus far and that my lupus was under control.

After turning twenty-four years old, I saw Dr. Lawrence on July 7, 1976 and everything was still going well for me. Therefore, she told me to start taking half of a 5 mg Prednisone pill daily. After being on that small amount of Prednisone everyday, I never experienced any pain at all. In September, my left foot was causing me some pain again. It felt like there was always something pulling in my veins. It could have been due to the type of shoes I was wearing.

When October came, I was still feeling the pulling sensation in my foot. I was having more nosebleeds as well.

On November 10, 1976, I had a clinic appointment with Dr. Lawrence. She let me know that everything so far was doing alright. She also said that my blood tests were in the controlled stage, but not fully cured. I told Dr. Lawrence about the pain that I was having in my left foot. She told me that it was okay and there was nothing serious to worry about. I was not experiencing any joint pains from my lupus and no new developments had occurred. I was currently taking half of a 5 mg Prednisone pill daily. Dr. Lawrence advised me to start taking my pills a little differently: From November 10th to December 1, 1976, I would be taking half of a 5 mg Prednisone pill daily, except on Saturdays. Beginning December 2nd to February 23, 1977, I would be taking half of a 5 mg Prednisone pill daily, except for

Tuesdays and Saturdays. On April 13, 1977, I would have to take blood and urine tests. Then, I would see Dr. Lawrence again on April 20th. That was going to be at least a five-month long test without seeing her.

Dr. Lawrence had been trying to get me off all Prednisone medication—slowly, but surely. I was not even taking any more iron pills. I was hoping that at my next clinic visit, everything would continue to improve for me.

Secretarial Position Has Ended

After about eight months of service working with the Juvenile Diabetes Foundation, they had to eliminate my position as full time secretary due to a limited budget and a very small staff. They tried to find another spot for me within the organization, but it was just not possible. Upon leaving, I was given a very nice letter of recommendation. I really enjoyed having the privilege of working with such a great Foundation.

Time to Look for Another job

On December 8, 1976, it was a very cold and blustering day outside. I was on my way to the New York State Unemployment Office, in the Bronx New York. I had curlers on under my hat due to the nasty weather we were having outside. While I was at the Unemployment Office, I was informed that they had a position available that fit my qualifications. It was with The General Contractors Association. I really did not think that there were going to be any jobs available at that time. Plus, I was definitely not prepared to go on that interview knowing that I was wearing curlers under my hat. I had to go because the company was very anxious to see me that day. After I received the directions, I was on my way to the job.

When I arrived at The General Contractors Association, there were also two other young ladies—pretty much the same age as myself—waiting to be seen to interview for the exact same position. Mr. Mattson, who was the one doing the hiring, explained that he would be giving us a letter that must be completed in whatever shorthand style we used. He said that he would be looking for neatness, spelling, and accuracy.

The other two ladies and I began talking to one another once he left the room. I asked the two girls, "Who wants this job?" We all looked at each other. I told them that I definitely did not want the job because I had just signed up for unemployment. I also told them that, since I was wearing curlers under my hat, I would not be hired. Realizing that it was just between the two of them, they looked at each other and smiled.

When the interview process was ready to begin, one of the girls was called into the office. After she took the test, she came out shaking her head at us as she was leaving. That let us know that she did not do well on the test. Then, the second girl was called in for her interview. When she came out, she shook her head at me. She was the one, out of all three of us, that really wanted this job. I said to her, "Oh no…that leaves me!" When I was called, I felt a little nervous as I proceeded to the office. After Mr. Mattson administered the test to me, he just sat looking at me. He could surely see that my hat was looking very bulky with those big curlers under it. He politely asked, "Do you always wear curlers to an interview?"

"Definitely not!" I responded with a smile. I told him that since the weather was so bad outside, I did not want my hair to get all messed up. All he could do was just look at me and smile.

"Well your letter was done beautifully and your short-hand skills were top notch." He complimented. Mr. Mattson said that he would like to hire me and I would be working in his legal department.

"Legal department! I don't know a thing about legal work." I said.

"Are you a good speller?" He asked.

"Yes! That is definitely one of my greatest strengths." I answered. Mr. Mattson said that, since I liked spelling, he would be more than willing to train me to become a great legal secretary. He said that the test he gave me was perfect, with no misspelled words. He also said that my letter was clean looking and that it was perfectly and professionally styled. I was glad to hear that. Mr. Mattson told me that I would do well as a legal secretary and asked if I would be able to start working immediately. I was not at all excited, but he seemed like such a nice person to work for, that I could not let him down. I thought to myself, *This nice man wants me to be his legal secretary, without any legal experience, and is willing to train me... I better take the job!* And I did just that!

Working for The General Contractors Association of New York, Inc.

When I arrived at the GCA, Mr. Mattson was anxiously awaiting and happy to see me. He started introducing me to all of the staff, and everyone seemed to be very friendly. Plus, I loved the family atmosphere of the job. After meeting everyone, the employees told me that he was bragging about me, so they could not wait to meet me. I was surprised to hear them say that. Everyone made me feel so at ease and I knew that I was going to love working there. Furthermore, I was also quite happy to hear that I would be able to choose the hours that I would like to work, plus get an hour for lunch. They told me that, if I am with the company for one year, I would be entitled to one month paid vacation as well as twelve sick days per year. At the age of twenty-four, who wouldn't want to have a beautiful job like this! At that time, I was not having any problems with my health and I was off to a good start in this new chapter of my life.

A few months in, my job was in need of a reception-ist. Since they were so pleased with my work and I got along well with everyone, I told Mary, who was the Office Manager, that my sister, Claudette, was not working and would definitely be interested. So, after speaking with her, my sister came in for an interview and she was hired.

Could I Be Pregnant?

During the month of April, I noticed that my period had not come. It was not uncommon for me to miss a period and usually it didn't bother me when I missed. But something about missing it in April seemed just a little different to me. I told my husband, but he did not believe me. So, I went to Jacobi Hospital for a pregnancy test. I was told that the results of all pregnancy tests for all patients would be posted on the hospital's bulletin board as either *Negative or Positive.* They said after a few days, all I would have to do was come in and see my name on the results list.

Jacobi Hospital - My Results Were In

Robert went to Jacobi hospital to find out my results. He called me at my workplace. Claudette transferred the call to my office. I was anxious to hear the results of my test. Robert informed me that my results were posted on the bulletin board in the screening clinic of the hospital according to my chart number. He said that the results were listed as positive. Robert was not at all happy. He was terrified and did not want anyone to know. All he kept saying was, "I am not ready to have a child!" To hear him say that was so hurtful. *He sure wanted the first pregnancy that we lost and now, a few years later, he cannot handle this!* I thought to myself.

At that point in my life, I did not even care what he was thinking. All I knew was that I was so happy for that second pregnancy. I had a very stable job as a legal secretary, that I really enjoyed, and I always liked to save money. Plus, Robert's job was also stable. So, between the two of us, money was never an issue—even from the time we started dating. So, I did not understand what his problem was.

As long as I knew in my heart that I was mentally and physically ready to have a baby, I was going to have the baby with or without him! What was so amazing to me was, no matter what I was going through, I was feeling so excited and content that I did not want anything to go wrong with that pregnancy. My lupus had not been affecting me and I was not experiencing any kind of ailments. I knew that it was God's way of telling me that I was healthy, mature, and ready to have this baby. That was one of the happiest times of my life!

Married Life Was Suffering

One Sunday, I felt constantly aggravated by my husband. It came to the point where we just argued about everything. It was definitely not good for my health or the baby that I was carrying. I just could not take it anymore. My father told me that being under that kind of stress was not good for me or my baby. He also told me that I could come over to their house and stay until things cooled off. I thought about what my dad had said. I took some of my things and went to their house.

After staying away for three weeks, things seemed to have calmed down. So, I decided to return back home. Robert told me that he realized he was definitely wrong, and he should be proud that his wife was having his baby. He said that he was sorry, and he did not want anything to go wrong with the pregnancy.

Sharing the Good News with Dr. Lawrence

On April 20, 1977, I had a clinic appointment to see Dr. Lawrence. I shared the good news with her and she was so happy that I was pregnant. The first thing that she said to me was, "Valerie, are you going to name the baby after me?" I was very surprised to hear her say that! I just looked at her and smiled. She then told me that she was just kidding, but it certainly gave me something to think about. She told me that my lupus was doing very well and that she saw no reason why I would not be able to go the full nine months of my pregnancy without any complications. She told me to make sure that I take iron and prenatal vitamins.

I Have an Infection

During that next month—May—I was having some terrible pains in my side. It felt like it was in my tubes. I was getting so worried that I could be pregnant in my tubes. I also began to get a very bad rash on the lips of my vagina and was experiencing a lot of discharge. Urinating burned me so bad that I wanted to scream. So, on Thursday, May 17, 1977, my husband took me to Emergency at Misericordia Hospital. There was a Chinese doctor who examined me and said that I had a Monilia infection. He said that it was particularly common in pregnant women. He gave me a prescription for Monistat Cream, to be inserted inside and outside of the vaginal area. It took about a week and a half before the infection and the burning went away, and then everything cleared up nicely for me.

My New OB/GYN Doctor

Dr. Lawrence was the one who recommended my new OB/GYN, Dr. Samuel Oberlander, to me. She also updated him on my history of lupus. After meeting with Dr. Oberlander, he was such a pleasant person that I immediately felt at ease. I was so excited to hear my baby's heartbeat for the very first time. Dr. Oberlander said that everything was going to be fine and that my delivery date would be December 10, 1977. My weight was 125 pounds. He gave me a prescription for Ferrous Gluconate (an Iron supplement) and Stuart Natal vitamins.

When I had a clinic appointment with Dr. Lawrence on June 1, 1977, she told me that my lupus was doing fine. She wanted me to decrease my Prednisone pills. She said that on Mondays, I did not need to take any Prednisone pills. On Tuesdays, I should take half of a 5 mg Prednisone pill. On Wednesdays, I did not need to take anything. On Thursdays, I should take half of a 5 mg Prednisone pill. On Fridays, I did not need to take anything. On Saturdays, I should take half of a 5 mg Prednisone pill, and on Sundays, I should take half of a 5 mg Prednisone pill. I was also taking, at the request of my OB/GYN, one Stuart Natal vitamin daily and three Ferrous Gluconate Iron pills daily.

I had an appointment with Dr. Oberlander on July 5, 1977; I was twenty-five years old. After the doctor measured my stomach, I was able to hear the baby's heartbeat. The doctor told me that the baby's heartbeat sounded strong and that the baby was growing very well. I saw Dr. Lawrence at the Arthritis Clinic the next day.

My Doctor Was Leaving

July 6, 1977 was the day that my doctor broke the news to her patients that she was leaving the Arthritis Clinic and would be taking on a new position as Director of Hematology. I felt so hurt by the news. Dr. Lawrence was such a caring doctor to me through the years and I could not believe that she was leaving. She told me not to worry. She said that everything was going to go very well for me. She advised me to continue decreasing my Prednisone medication as instructed by the new doctor. She also told me that, in the event that anything should go wrong with me, she can always be reached at the hospital.

Dr. Lawrence had been with me from the most crucial time in my life to the most gratifying—when she learned of my becoming a mother. She has given so much of herself, and I am truly grateful for everything she has done for me. She advised that on Mondays, I should not take anything. On Tuesdays, I should take half of a 5 mg Prednisone pill. On Wednesdays, I should not take anything. On Thursdays, I should take half of a 5 mg Prednisone pill. On Fridays, I should not take anything. On Saturdays, I should take half of a 5 mg Prednisone pill. On Sundays, I should not take anything. I continued to take three Ferrous Gluconate iron pills daily and one Stuart Natal vitamin daily.

August 17, 1977 was the first clinic appointment

that I had with my new doctor. His name was Dr. Kalish. Dr. Kalish informed me that after looking over my hospital records, my health was doing fine and there was nothing for me to worry about.

I saw Dr. Kalish for the second time on October 12, 1977. After taking some blood and urine tests everything came back fine. I could not believe how well my pregnancy was going and I was not experiencing any problems. Then, I saw Dr. Kalish on November 9, 1977. I was near to the end of my pregnancy and everything was going okay.

When I had an appointment with Dr. Oberlander, I told him that I was getting a lot of cramps in my hips and it slowed me down a great deal when I walked. Dr. Oberlander said that it was normal and that there was nothing to worry about. He also informed me that the baby was resting on my muscles, which was causing that terrible pain for me. Another thing that was happening to me, was that my feet would start swelling at around 12:00 Noon and stay that way into the night. Other than that, I did not have any other problems.

After I visited with Dr. Oberlander, I really started thinking about everything. I had been feeling so heavy and weighted down. I had been climbing the stairs and taking the train back and forth to work everyday, and it started taking a toll on me. My weight was 157 pounds. Since I was near to the end of my pregnancy, on November 14, 1977 I decided to stop working. On Tuesdays, I was taking half of a 5 mg Prednisone pill. On Thursdays, I was taking half of a 5 mg Prednisone pill, and on Saturdays, I was taking half of a 5 mg Prednisone pill.

I informed Dr. Oberlander that it seemed like I was not feeling the baby as much. The movements of the baby had slowed down quite a bit and were not like they were in my earlier months of the pregnancy. So, he had me take a test to see how the baby would react. That took about three hours to complete and kept making the baby jump. I was informed that all of the results were okay and that there was nothing to worry about.

I Was in Labor

Two weeks later, I started having contractions. The contractions started on December 12, 1977, about 7:00 AM, and they were about thirty minutes apart. Then, about 3:00 PM, they were fifteen minutes apart. By 6:00 PM, the pain was five minutes apart. We called Dr. Oberlander. He had another doctor call me back to let me know what I should do. Dr. Oberlander's standby doctor told me to come straight to the hospital. So, we did. When we arrived, the doctor gave me an internal examination. He said the baby would not be born until midnight, or maybe early that next morning. The doctor advised us to go back home. He gave me a 100 mg Pentobarbital Capsule to help relieve the pain a little.

After I returned home, I drank some hot tea, but nothing seemed to soothe me or help to make the pain any better for me. About 8:30 PM, which was not long after I got home, I had to rush back to the doctor because the pain was now only a minute apart. The doctor kept me in the hospital, but he said that my baby was still not ready. I did stay overnight like the doctor predicted. Robert stayed with me while I was in labor. He left when the pains got worse. At around 8:30 that next morning—on December 13, 1977—Dr. Oberlander rushed into my room. He told me, "Valerie, I'm taking the baby now because you're suffering too long."

Then, he broke my water. He advised that I would have the baby naturally. The anesthesiologist inserted a needle into my spine. She said that it would numb me from the waist down and it did. Then, they called my husband. When Robert arrived, they were rushing me into the delivery room—about something to nine in the morning. Robert was able to hear everything that was going on. The doctor kept telling me to push harder and harder. I did not know how or what the heck I was pushing. I knew I had broken a lot of blood vessels. The doctor did not have to use any forceps. Before I knew it, my baby was being born.

My Baby Was Born

My little baby girl was born on December 13, 1977 at 9:12 AM at Albert Einstein College of Medicine in the Bronx, New York. She weighed 7 lbs. 14½ oz. and was 20½ inches long. I was told that my little girl had jaundice and was being put under the lights for observation. She also had her father's blood type.

I thought a lot about it, and I was truly honored to give my little girl my doctor's full name. I did in fact name my little girl Christine. I used my doctor's last name to give my baby Lauren as her middle name. That worked out so well. Her full name is Christine Lauren Horn.

While I was in the delivery room, the first thing they showed me were her first footprints. When they wheeled me into the recovery room, I could feel my insides contracting back. My urine had stopped, my bowel movements stopped, and my throat was so sore. I could not even swallow anything and I was so thirsty. The hospital assigned two student helpers to assist in whatever I needed. That was so thoughtful of the hospital to do that for me.

When they brought me back to the ward, I was really in bad shape (i.e.: stitches, catheter to help me urinate, and an IV in my arm.) I lost so much blood, that I was given three blood transfusions. They took several blood and urine tests to see what was going on with me. I was too sick to even hold my own baby. When my baby looked at me as they rolled her into my room, that made me keep reliving the terrible pain that I experienced. I kept asking myself, *That baby came out of me?*

After a little time had passed, and I was still in the hospital a few days before Christmas, I was told that I had a Hematoma—a collection of blood outside of the blood vessel. I was told that a slight operation would have to be performed. I signed papers authorizing the operation. The operation was done on a Saturday and it was very successful. While I was in the recovery room after the operation, the surgeon told me that I had blood clots inside of me that were 'as big as oranges.' He also said that there were some more blood clots inside of me that would eventually come out as soon as my period came back again. The doctor packed me inside with gauze and a tube was put inside of me to drain the excess blood out.

On Christmas morning, the nurse brought my little baby girl into my room. While I started to undress her, her navel dropped off. I started talking to my baby by saying, "Christine, look at how long we've been in this hospital together!" I said Merry Christmas to my little baby girl. All of my family was there visiting with us. I was very happy to see everyone. My oldest brother Alonzo (stepbrother) and his wife Janice gave me two nice brass trinkets to put on the Christmas tree when we got home. One trinket was with our baby's name and birth date written on it, and the other one had, "Horn Family" written on it. I appreciated that very much because it was unique.

On December 27, 1977, the doctor decided to take my packing out early that morning before breakfast was served. That procedure was very, very painful. The following day on December 28th, the doctor removed the tube that was inserted in me, as well as the stitches. After all of that was done, the doctor said that I could finally leave the hospital that same day. I immediately called Robert. After Robert arrived, the doctor informed us that our little baby would not be coming home with us. The doctor said that they would like to watch her for just one more day. So, my husband and I were feeling sad that we had to leave without our baby. I had been through so much already since she was born.

December 29, 1977 was the day that my husband and

I got to pick up our little baby girl from the hospital. We were both so relieved that our little girl was doing well, and we were finally happy to have her home with us. That was definitely an exciting year! I thought to myself and looked forward to the beginning of another New Year.

I had a doctor's appointment on January 25, 1978 at the Arthritis Clinic. Dr. Kalish said that everything was fine. I was not having any joint pains or anything. I dropped a good amount of weight after having my baby and I weighed in at 130 pounds.

My Six Week Checkup With My OB/GYN

Around 2:00 AM, I started getting very bad pains in my stomach and on my left side. I could not even stand up straight. Since the pain was so unbearable, I decided to take two Anacin tablets. About 4:00 AM, Robert and I decided we would go to the hospital, but the pain did seem to have subsided a little. When I got into the car, I started feeling much better, so we decided it wasn't worth rushing to the hospital. Then, at around 8:00 AM, when the Anacin tablets completely wore off, the pain came back. I took a taxi to see Dr. Oberlander for my six-week checkup since Robert had already left for work. Dr. Oberlander began checking me internally. It was so painful that he decided to admit me into the hospital. With all the signs that I was having, the doctors thought that it could be my appendix and said that it may have to be removed. They immediately took some x-rays and blood tests, but found nothing wrong. My doctor had me stay in the hospital for another two days just in case something else developed.

Robert explained to the doctors that, when he was young, he had to have his appendix taken out because that was "life or death." He further told the doctors, "Since y'all don't know exactly what it is, I think y'all should wait!"

When the next day came, I woke up that morning and all the pain had already gone away. My stomach did not even hurt when the doctors pressed on it. That was a very good sign for me. The doctors were so amazed and could not even believe what was happening. Robert said, "You see, they would have taken your appendix out for nothing!" The doctors said it was probably my period trying to come on. I was then discharged. My period came on March 4, 1978.

I had an appointment to see Dr. Kalish at the Arthritis Clinic on March 8, 1978. I explained to Dr. Kalish that sometime in February, I noticed that my left hip was starting to feel a little achy. He said that a lot of lupus patients tend to have that problem. He suggested that I get some x-rays taken on my next visit with him, which would be on April 5th. In the meantime, he had me stop all Prednisone pills the last two weeks in March.

Christine's Ears Were Being Pierced

When it was April 1, 1978, my baby girl, Christine, was almost four-months old when I took her to get her little tiny ears pierced. My sister Vanessa's sister-in-law, Norma, was gracious enough to do the procedure, and my little girl's tiny gold earrings looked so cute in her ears.

Doctors Appointments at the Arthritis Clinic

On April 5th, Dr. Kalish was unable to make it to my Arthritis Clinic appointment in time for my x-rays to be taken because of some car trouble he was having. Therefore, I was unable to have my x-rays done. He did arrive at 10:30 AM, but I had already left with my husband and daughter. I was still off all Prednisone medication.

On June 7, 1978, when I was at my clinic appointment at Jacobi Hospital, Dr. Kalish told me that I was doing great after having my daughter. I knew it was due to the gradual decreasing of my Prednisone that made my lupus less likely to flare-up.

Job Anxious for Me to Come Back!

My boss at the GCA started calling me, trying to find out when, and if, I would be returning back to work after maternity leave. My life with Robert was not going good at all. I decided that since my job kept calling me, and really wanted me to come back, that I better get myself back to work. Therefore, I had to look for a good day care center to put my little girl in. I had serious thoughts about leaving my husband.

I had a clinic appointment with my doctor on June 25, 1978. My doctor said that everything was doing fine. I did not have any joint pains.

Time to Separate

On July 3, 1978, on my way home from work, I had to pick up my little girl from Memo's Day Care Center. It was an excellent day care. When I returned home and opened the door to my apartment, I started looking through my hall closet to find the outfit that I wanted to wear for the 4th of July holiday. I was looking forward to going out with my friends, since Robert never seemed to want to go out anywhere as a married couple.

Robert was not home at the time, but I noticed that the outfit I was supposed to be wearing tomorrow was ripped and the buttons were torn off. I could not believe what I was seeing! I was hot like fire! He didn't even want to go out with me; so why would he rip my clothes? How jealous and crazy was that? I could not and would not stay in the apartment with him any longer. It was just too abusive. My first priority was my child and I did not want to subject her to that. A child should always be in a healthy environment and that was not it. It was time for my seven-month-old daughter and I to leave!

I was twenty-six years old when I separated. I was spending time figuring things out. What was so amazing to me was, when Robert and I were dating, we would see each other on the weekends and always looked forward to spending quality time with family and friends. Once we got married everything changed. As far as our goals were concerned, we were definitely not headed in the same direction.

My little girl, that I love so much, has truly been a blessing to me. She was the one that gave me all the strength and the courage that I needed to keep moving forward. I planned to come back and get all of the furniture and the rest of our things once I got situated in a place of my own.

Christine's Christening Day

On the morning of November 26, 1978, my family and I were at Crawford Methodist Church in the Bronx, New York. It was Christine Lauren Horn's Christening Day. She was eleven months old. That morning she was so irritable that she just cried and cried. The rest of our day was well spent at my parent's house with our family and friends.

Recouping My Belongings

After only a short period of time after leaving Robert, I was able to find a very nice place to live. It just happened to be right around the corner from where my parents were living. It was time for me to recoup all of my belongings.

Well, during the morning of my move, I instructed the movers to take all of the furniture out of the apartment, as well as roll up all of the carpets off of the floors. Robert did, however, keep his stereo that he loved so much, as well as a few pots and pans. After taking everything that I needed, I knew that Robert was not going to be able to stay in that lonely empty apartment all by himself. I was so glad that my move was going smoothly. When the movers were ready to pull off, I suddenly realized that I left my keys to the new apartment upstairs in my hall closet.

I had to slowly tip-toe back upstairs and get the keys off the top shelf of the hall closet without my husband seeing me. As I began walking back up the stairs, I could hear the pots and pans and music playing. He was in the kitchen. My closet door could be seen from the reflection of the mirrors from the kitchen. I slowly opened the door and felt for my keys on the top shelf of the closet. I reached for them and he heard me.

"What are you doing?" he asked.

"I left my keys." I said before hurrying back down the stairs. As the movers were ready to pull away, Robert got into his car and followed behind us.

When we arrived, Robert was surprised to see that I was renting an apartment in a two family house—which was right around the corner from where my parents were living. He was pleased. He helped me with some of my things and was hoping that one day we would get back together. My landlord had already been informed of my situation, and I tried my best to stay as calm as possible so that there would not be any conflict. After that, Robert told me that he was headed back to the apartment, but would eventually be moving out. I told him to make sure he gives the landlord advance notice. I was finally happy to be at peace.

My health had been doing pretty well that following year, and I did not experience any lupus flare-ups. I had also moved forward with my divorce.

Taking the Post Office Exam - 1980

I always liked looking through the Chief Newspaper to see which jobs would be coming available. So, on May 12, 1980, I took the Mail Handler Post Office Exam in Flushing, New York. I liked keeping my options open, so I decided to take the exam. On June 26, 1980, the day before my birthday, I was informed that I passed the exam with a final rating of 89.4 and it was entered on the register as eligible. On November 4, 1980 I had been offered a temporary position which included night work. My daughter was very young and I could not accept working at night. Therefore, I kept my current job—that I still loved—which was full time, more secure, and not temporary.

Thanksgiving Trip to Greensboro, North Carolina

During Thanksgiving weekend of 1980, I decided to take a trip with my friend, Charles, to visit with his relatives. When we were driving down, Charles, Christine, and I were all sitting in the back seat of the car for many hours. After that, I started experiencing a lot of joint pains. I did not know if I would even make it to North Carolina. I started taking some arthritis pain medication that I brought with me, just in case. It seemed to help.

Thank God that we were all able to arrive safely in Greensboro, North Carolina that Thanksgiving morning. As the day went on, and I was meeting everyone, I forgot all about the pain. The climate in North Carolina just seemed to have taken all of my pain away while I was there and my trip was a success.

Lupus Flare-up – I Have a New Doctor – 12/1980

When Christine and I arrived back home in New York that same week, I started getting sick. I also had an appointment with my doctor at the Arthritis Clinic. When I arrived, I was informed that Dr. Kalish who I was seeing for my lupus, had left the Arthritis Clinic and I had been assigned to a new doctor. Her name was Dr. Betty Diamond.

After meeting with Dr. Diamond that day, she saw that I was having a lupus flare-up. She said that my kidneys and joints were a major problem. Therefore, she immediately started me on twelve 5 mg Prednisone pills to avoid my lupus from getting way out of control. That was a total of 60 mgs of Prednisone daily. I did not like being on so much Prednisone medication because of the side effects. Dr. Diamond said that she believed in decreasing Prednisone pretty fast and that I would not be on it too long. That was so good to hear. She also had me on a 50 mg tablet of Hydrochlorothiazide.

My Husband Finally Withdraws His Answer

April 24, 1981 was a long time after I officially left Robert on July 4, 1978. Robert finally withdrew his answer and consented to my obtaining the divorce, as well as to paying child support. Robert had been stalling with the divorce papers, since I last filed in 1979 because he did not want the divorce. I thought to myself, "There must be a reason why he is anxious for the divorce to finally happen."

Dissolution of Marriage

"Hooray!" Less than a month later, my divorce became final. I was almost twenty-nine years old and was so glad that part of my life was finally over!

Off All Prednisone Medication

After all of the clinic visits that I had with Dr. Diamond, she was able to get me off all Prednisone medication. Everything was going fine. Even my blood pressure was back to normal and my weight was 135 pounds.

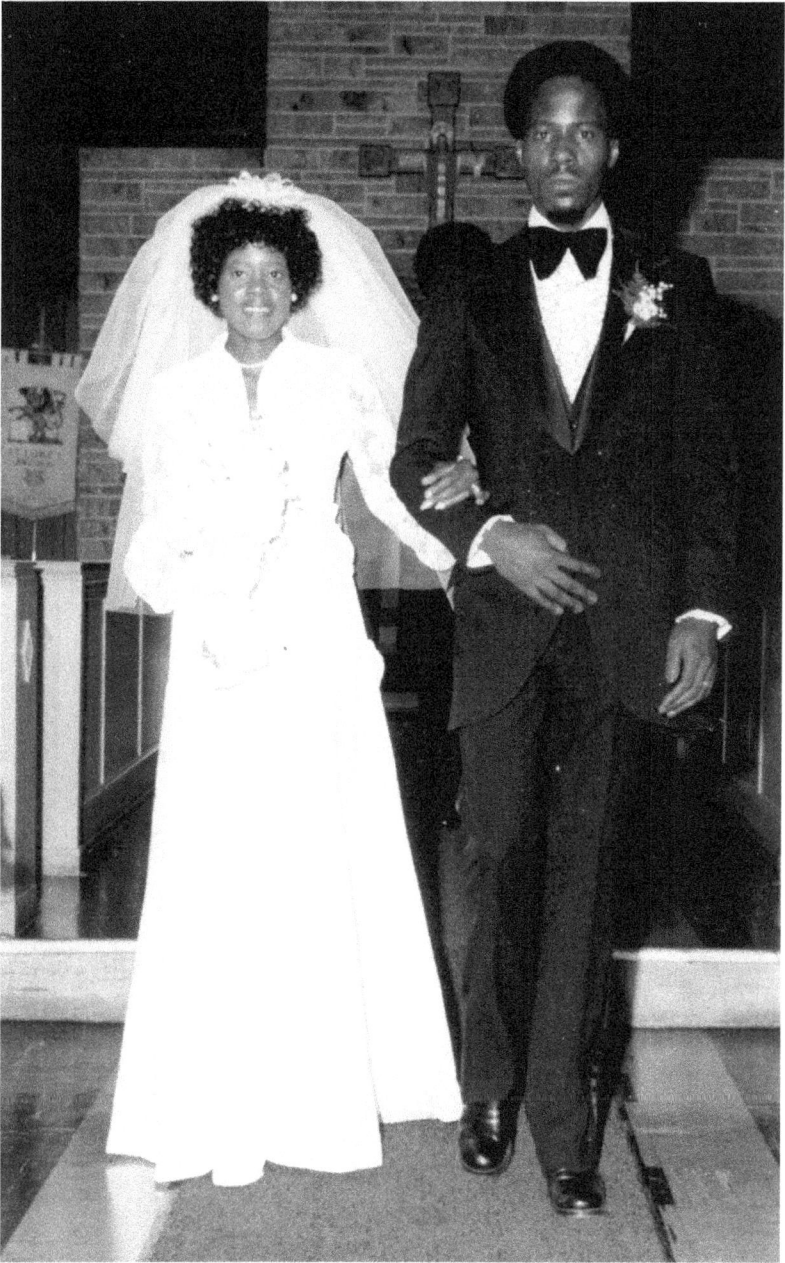

My Wedding Day - July 13, 1974
St. Luke's Episcopal Church

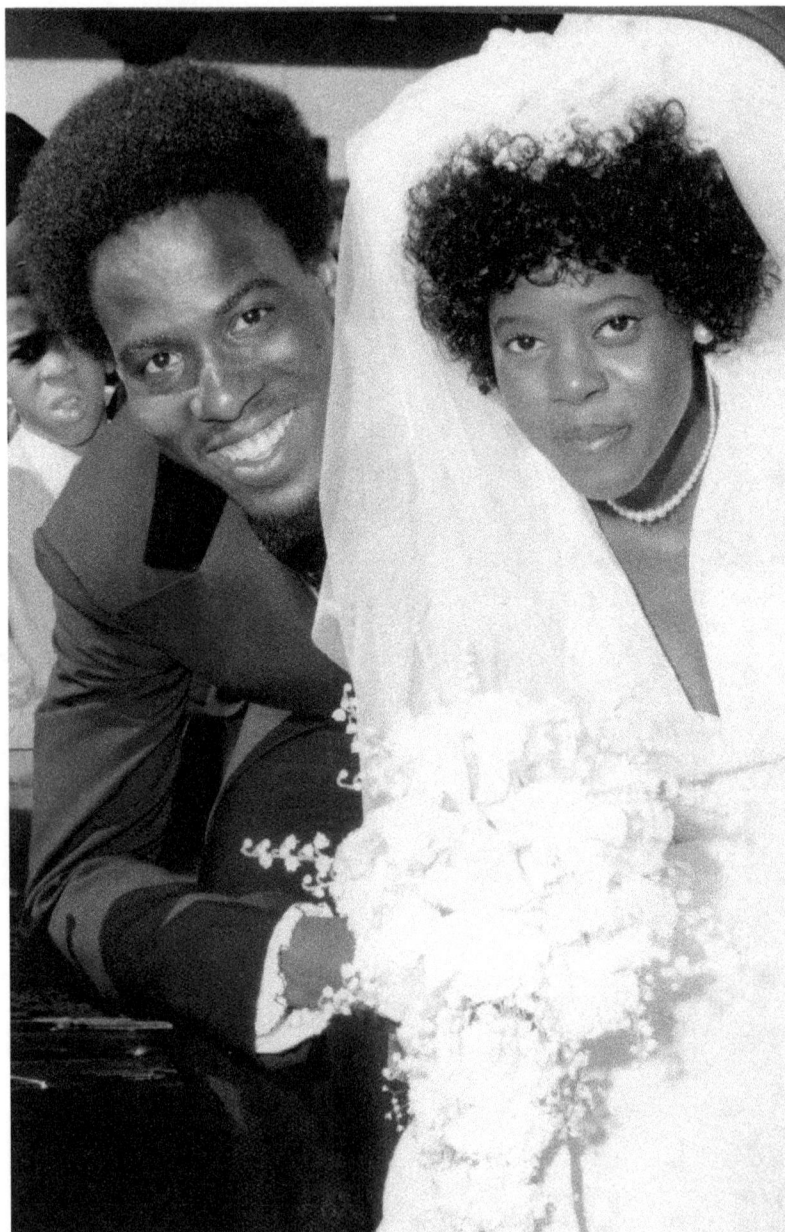

Left to right: My foster brother, Barry (background), and my husband and I.

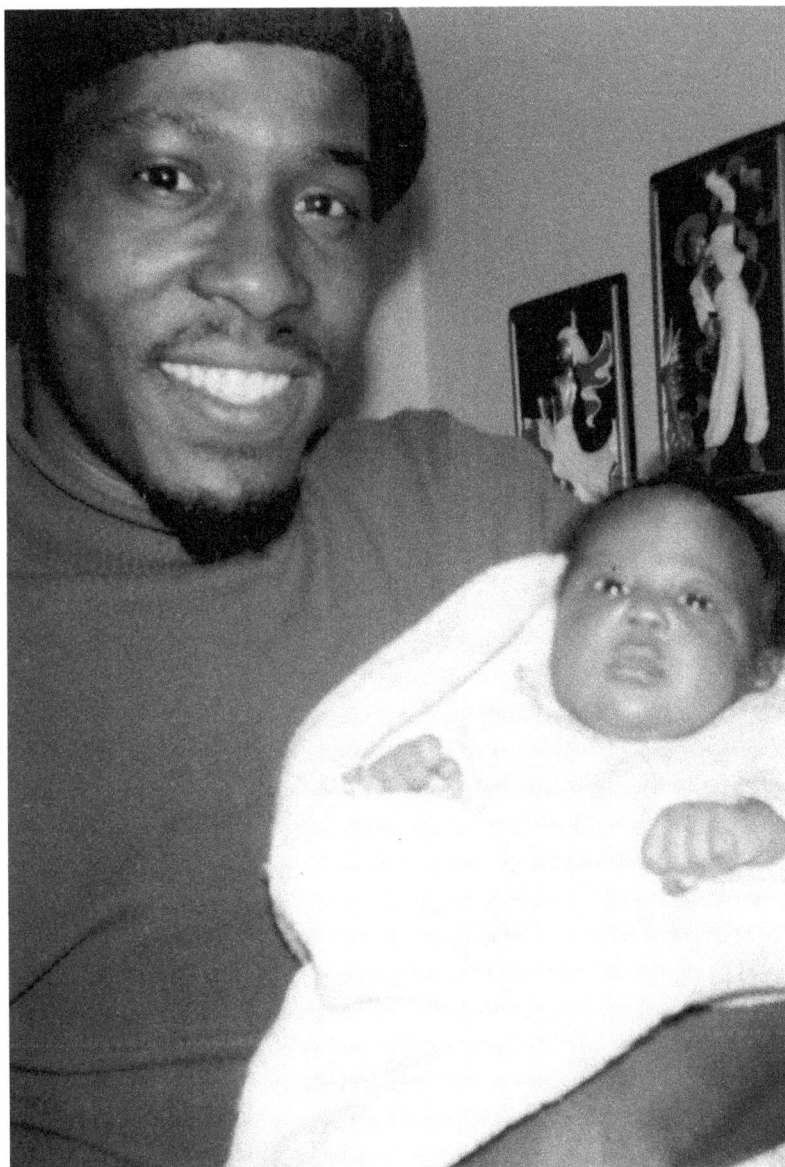

My husband and his daughter, Christine at home.

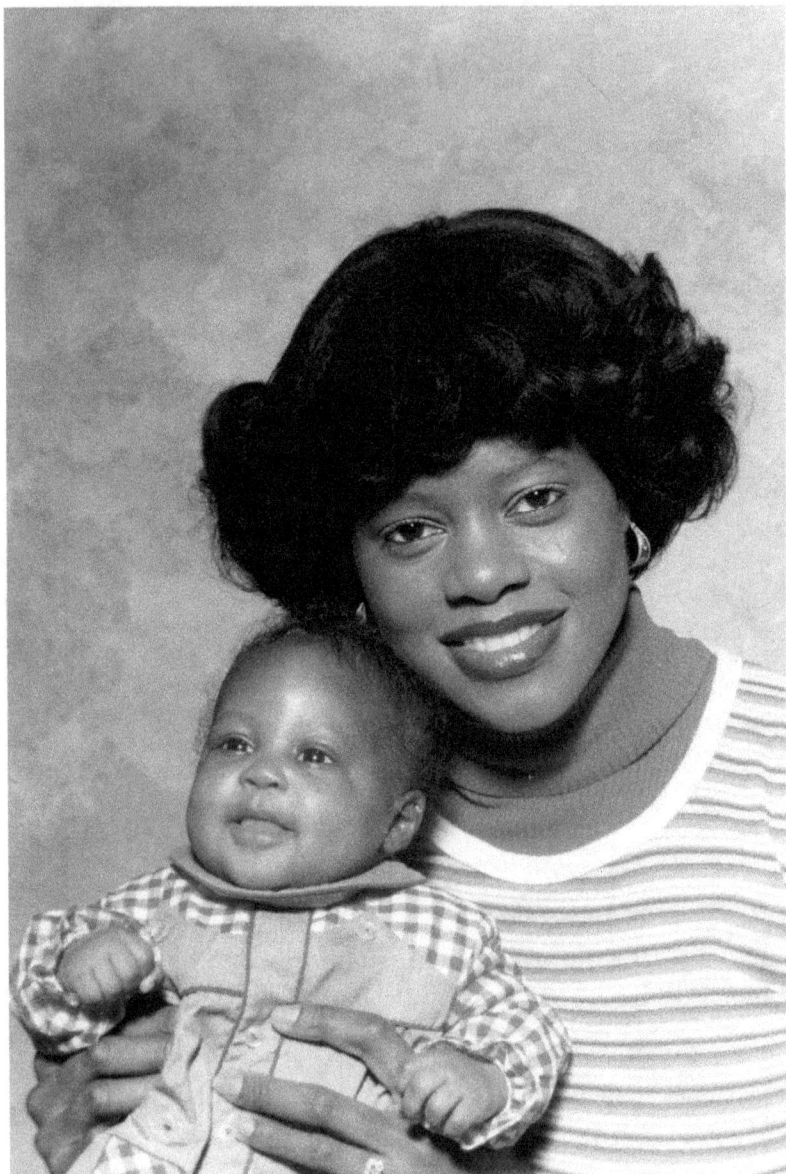

My daughter and I. Christine was six and a half weeks old.

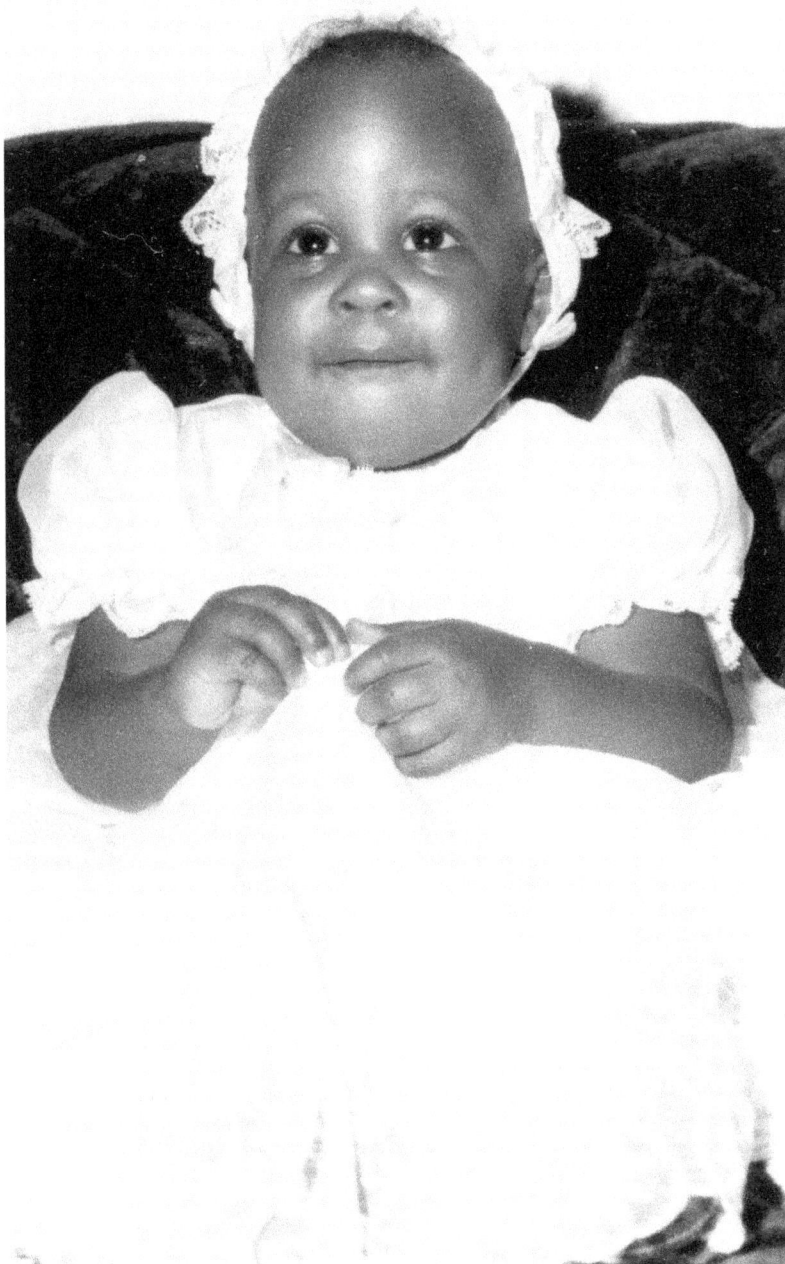

At my parent's house. Christine Lauren Horn's Christening Day -
November 26, 1978. She was eleven months old.

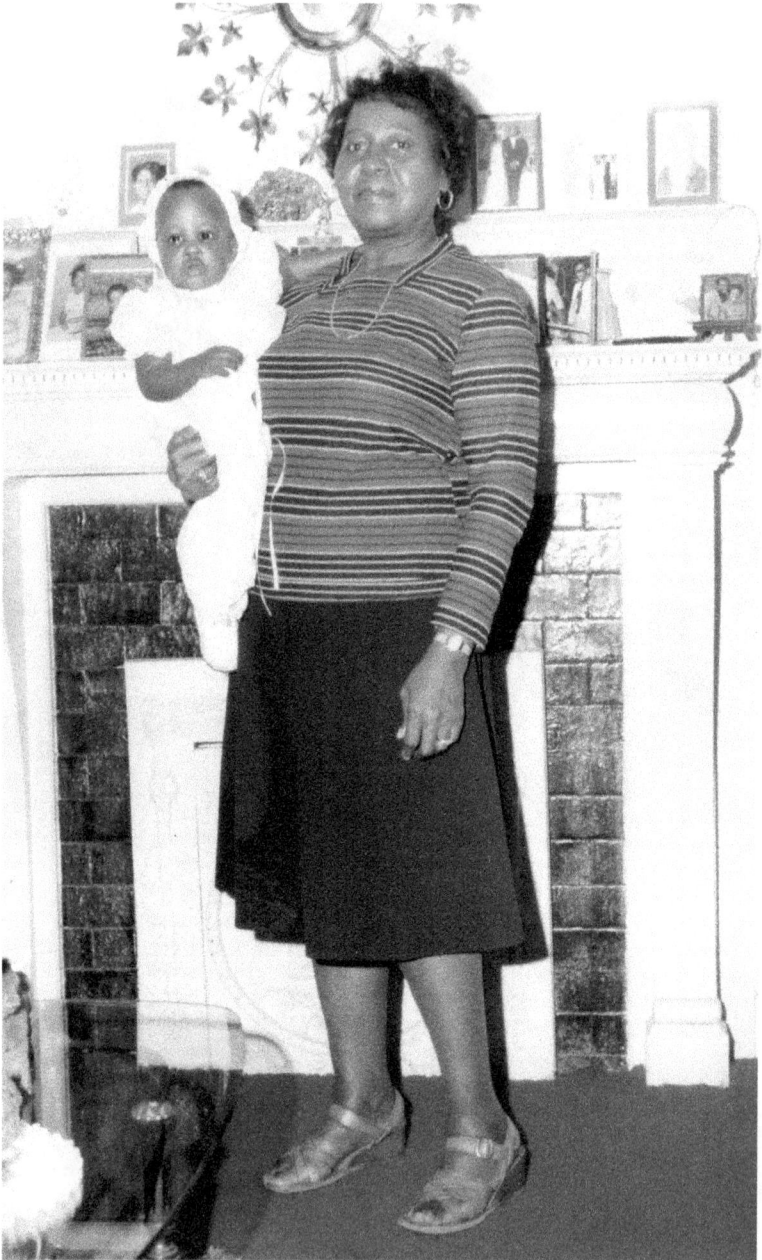

My daughter, and my mother - November 26, 1978.

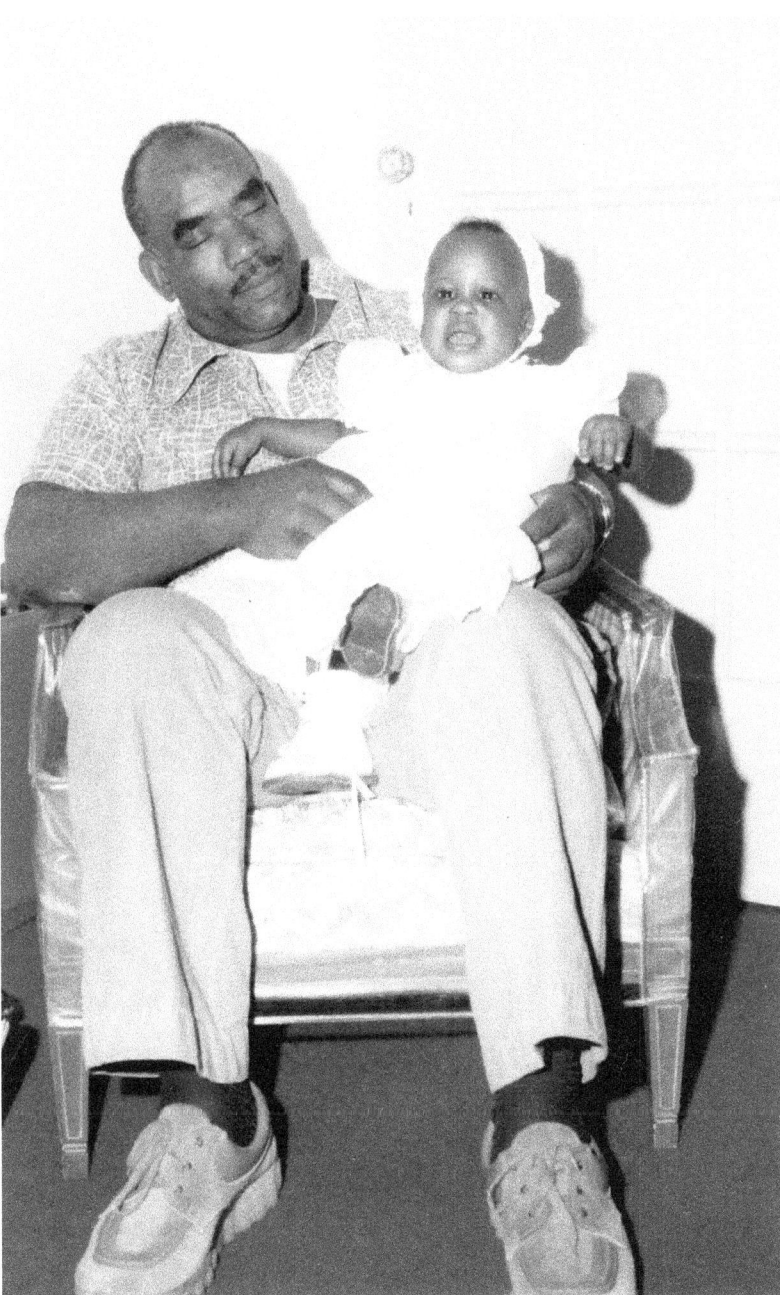

My stepfather, and my daughter - November 26, 1978.

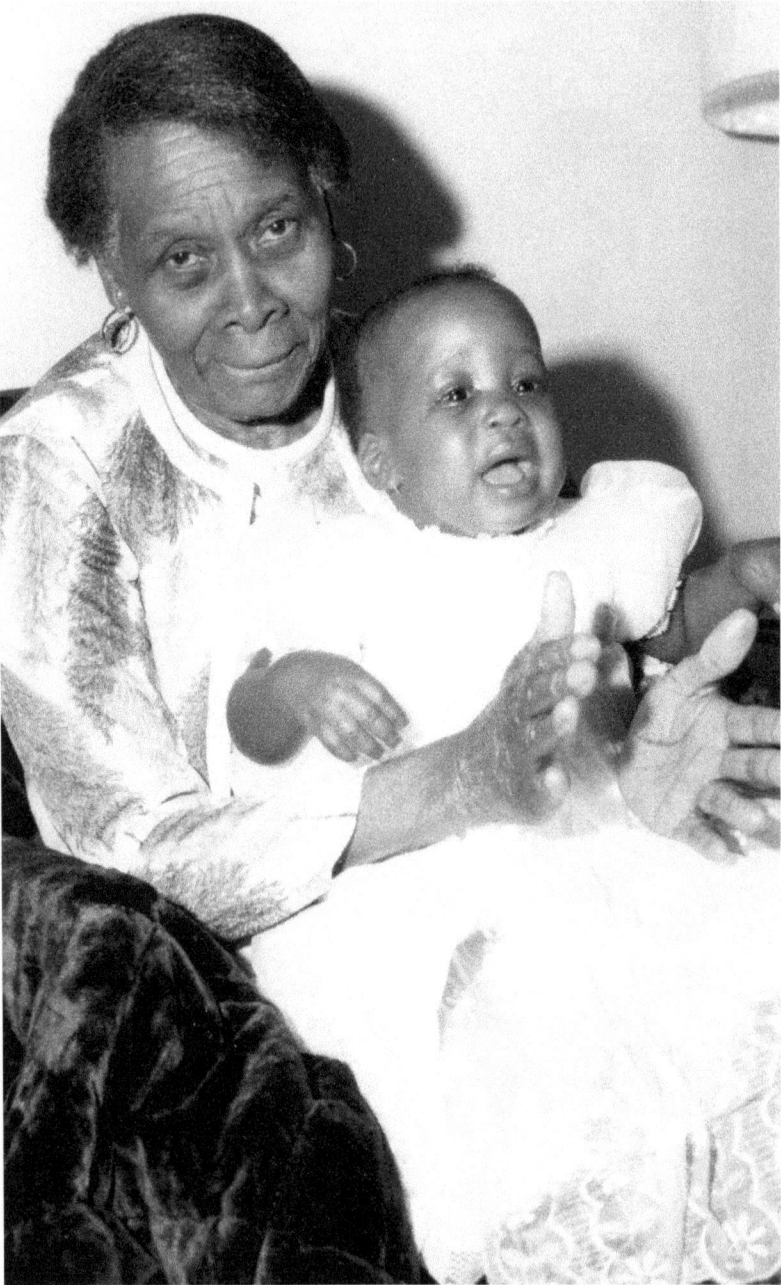

My grandmother was putting her hands together trying to soothe my daughter - November 26, 1978.

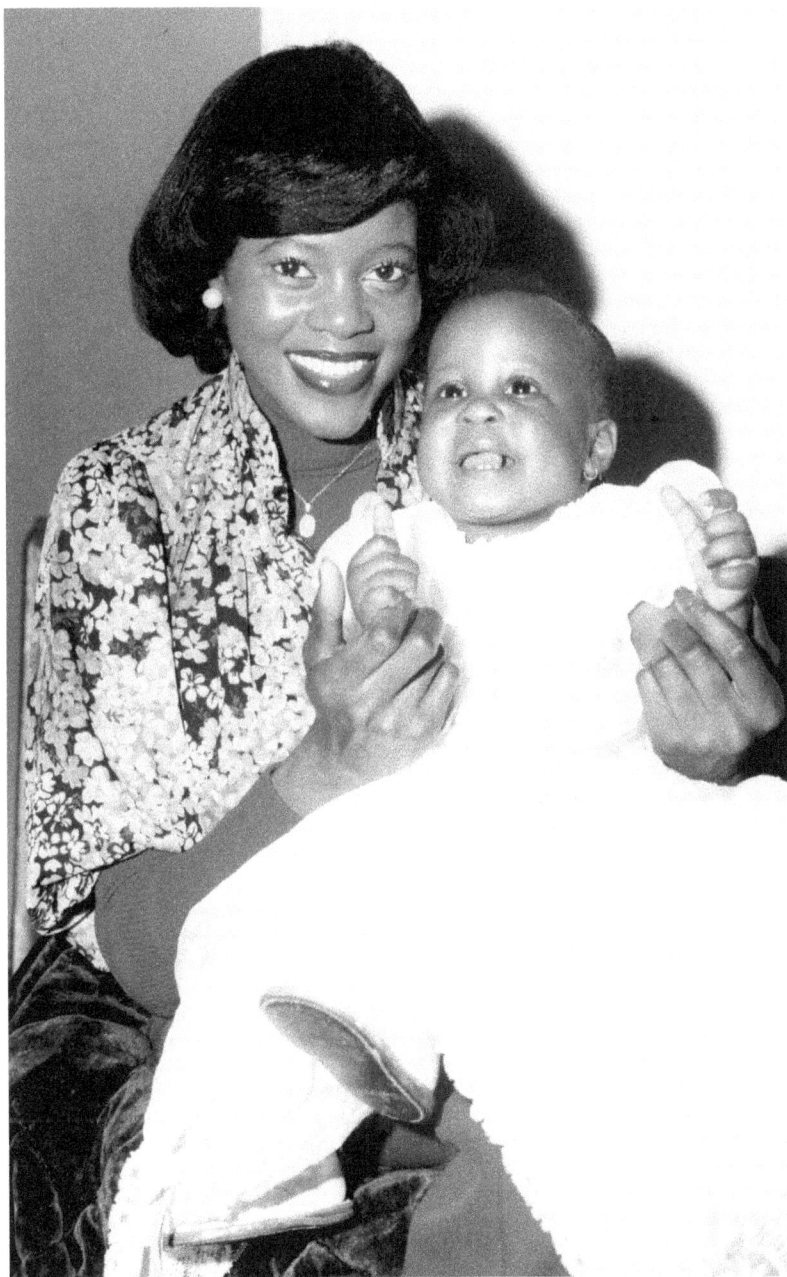
My daughter and I. She was quiet after I held her.

CHAPTER 4

LIFE AFTER DIVORCE

It was the beginning of the New Year in 1982, when I had another lupus flare-up. At that time, I was suffering with very severe pain in my left leg, near the thigh. I did not know what was going on, so I called my mother. When she came over, we immediately rushed to Jacobi Hospital.

We arrived at Jacobi Hospital's emergency room around 5:00 PM. The doctor in the emergency room did not waste any time and immediately gave me a shot in my thigh to relieve the severe pain I was experiencing. It helped a little. The doctors also checked my urine and the results showed that I was losing protein. Because I was also running a very high fever, they decided to admit me around midnight. After I was admitted into the ward, the doctors told me that the pain in my left leg would go away shortly, so they put some warm gauze around the painful area and continued to treat me with Tylenol with Codeine. It really helped me a lot. They quickly started an intravenous in my arm.

I had to stay in the hospital for a full week before the doctors could clear up my kidney infection. When I returned home, I continued to stay on Prednisone. Dr. Diamond rapidly decreased my Prednisone until I was completely off.

What Is This?

In February of 1982, I received a letter by mail to my new residence in the Bronx. It was a letter addressed to Robert from his health benefit plan. I thought to myself, *Why is he having his mail come to my new residence like he lives here? We are divorced!* I immediately notified him that he had mail. I thought that maybe it was our daughter's health benefits information, since they usually send that to me. Robert told me to open it. As I opened the letter, I was shocked! The letter was informing him that his "wife," Regina, was being added to his insurance policy—it showed her date of birth and the effective date of coverage.

I thought to myself, *Wife... He is not married.* This was the same person who sent a letter to my home when I was moving out. He thought the envelope was addressed to Mrs. Horn and not Mr. Horn. I knew exactly what it said, so I opened it. He told me that it was from a friend who was inviting him to her college graduation in Upstate New York. I did not care what it said and I gave it back to him.

I was so mad that he had the nerve to take his four-year-old daughter off of his medical coverage just so he could put his girlfriend on. Even though I had medical insurance through my employer, I could not believe he would do that. I finally found the answer I was looking for. He consented to the divorce because his girlfriend, not "wife," was pregnant. That letter was all the proof I needed.

Child Support Through Payroll Deduction

At the time, Robert and I were in court to have child support monies taken out. I had to do this because Robert was not paying child support and he was liable for the support of his daughter. Robert consented to everything, and on October 22, 1982, it became effective.

Lupus Flare-up - 2/22/83

When I had a clinic appointment on February 22, 1983, I was thirty years old and having a lupus flare-up. I had to start taking ten 5 mg Prednisone pills daily. I also noticed that my urine had become very bubbly, like soap. Dr. Diamond told me that it was due to a kidney infection. My kidneys had been losing protein and it was coming out in my urine. My ankles were still swelling, even after getting a full eight hours of sleep. I did not experience as much joint pain as I used to in my teen years. I also noticed that my kidneys were having repeated flare-ups once I reached my late twenties. I wished that Dr. Diamond could always keep me on a very small dose of Prednisone, so that I would not flare-up so fast, but I knew that was not possible. I did not like being on so much Prednisone when my lupus flared-up.

During March 16, 1983, we were having nice weather in New York City. I also had a clinic appointment at that time. I was on ten 5 mg Prednisone pills a day. Dr. Diamond decided that on Friday, March 18, 1983, I would decrease my Prednisone to eight 5 mg pills a day. Then, in two more weeks, I could decrease my Prednisone to six pills a day. Dr. Diamond prescribed a 50 mg Hydrochlorothiazide water pill to be taken daily for hypertension. She also decided to put me on a new medication called Imuran, which was a 50 mg pill to be taken once a day with my Prednisone. Dr. Diamond felt that, by taking two, maybe it would help the kidneys. She said that taking Prednisone alone was not really doing the job like it should for me.

I was still having bubbles in my urine, which was the main concern. By my next appointment in April, Dr. Diamond would be able to see what was going to happen from there. I was unable to see my doctor for our April 6th appointment.

My Doctor Said, "Something Has to Be Done."

I was thirty years old and meeting with Dr. Diamond at the Arthritis Clinic on April 27, 1983. There were no changes with the blood that was still in my urine. She felt that something had to be done about this problem. She suggested that a Cystoscopy examination be given to me at the hospital. She referred me to that department for an evaluation.

Then, on May 6, 1983, I met with the Cystoscopy department and they explained everything that they wanted to do. First, they felt that I should have x-rays taken of my bladder and kidneys—this was done by shooting some dye into the veins of my arm. That way, they would be able to detect if there were any cysts or something else that might be causing me to have the bubbles in my urine. They said that the test would be given to me that following Monday.

The next week, when I had all of those tests done, my x-rays were all negative even though I still had blood in my urine. So, on May 11th and May 25th I had appointments at the Arthritis Clinic to meet with Dr. Diamond. Still, nothing had changed.

Dr. Diamond referred me back to the third floor, once again, for further study and tests on July 1, 1983. After speaking with the Cystoscopy department, they suggested that I have the examination done that Friday, July 15th at 1:00 PM.

On July 6, 1983, I had an appointment at the Arthritis Clinic. At that time, I was thirty-one years old. Dr. Diamond mentioned that being on Prednisone and Imuran was not helping the problem that I was having. She said that it was going on for far too long and that something needed to be done immediately.

Cystoscopy Examination Done at Jacobi Hospital on 7/15/83

I was on my way to Jacobi Hospital on July 15, 1983;

the weather in New York City was extremely hot. It was 95 to 100 degrees. The doctor told me before the exam, that if they did not find out what was causing the blood in my urine they would have to admit me into the hospital for further testing. They said that would include having a biopsy done. I was not looking forward to that.

The Cystoscopy examination was done at 2:30 PM and it really hurt. They had to do the exam three times because the first two exams did not work. Well, believe it or not, the tests did not come out bad after all. The tests showed that I had inflammation of the Trigonitis. They said that, with antibiotics such as Bactrim, it would clear up in about five days.

After I took Bactrim for a solid month—which was around late August—it was supposed to clear up my kidneys, but it didn't do anything. I did not feel bad and was taken off all medications.

When I visited Dr. Diamond at the Arthritis Clinic on October 26th, I told her that nothing was currently bothering me. I could not believe that the bubbles in my urine had all disappeared. My urine tests were negative. Therefore, I did not have to see Dr. Diamond again until December 28th.

My Hair Was Falling Out

On the 11th of November, when I washed my hair, a big glob of it fell out. Then, on November 18th, when I washed my hair in the shower, all the roots of my hair came out and went down into the drain of the tub. I was really worried. Then, on November 25th, I went to the hairdresser so that she could see what was going on. I told her that I wasn't sure if it was my wool hat that was causing the hair loss or if it was a side effect of taking the new Imuran medication.

My hairdresser told me that the type of hat that I was wearing would not have caused my hair to come out like that. So, on December 2, 1983, I decided to call Dr. Diamond because my hair was falling out like crazy—roots and all. She informed me that Imuran does not have hair loss as a side effect. She told me to come to the clinic on December 7th because it could be a lupus flare-up.

Lupus Flare-up – 12/7/83

When I saw Dr. Diamond on December 7, 1983, she had me take some blood and urine tests. She said that she would get the results back while I waited. When the results were ready, it was confirmed that I was experiencing a lupus flare-up. She had to start me on three 5 mg pills of Prednisone a day. Dr. Diamond wanted to see me again before the year was out.

I saw Dr. Diamond on December 28th. I was reduced to two 5 mg pills of Prednisone a day. I felt fine, but my hair was still falling out a little bit. Dr. Diamond told me that being on two pills of Prednisone a day should clear up my hair trouble and that putting me on a high dose was really not necessary for that minor problem.

We entered into the New Year of 1984. On January 25th, I was seen at the Arthritis Clinic. All of my hair trouble had cleared up very nicely. Dr. Diamond told me to go down to one 5 mg Prednisone pill for another two weeks. Then, I could go completely off. She told me that if there was any slight change, to make sure and see her as soon as possible. She had me take urine and blood tests, and on March 28, 1984, I would get the results.

On March 28, 1984, when I saw Dr. Diamond, she informed me that, from all of the tests that I had taken, I needed to get back on Prednisone. I said to myself, *Here I go again!*

Discovering My Roots

Since my biological father died when I was just a little girl, I felt that it was time to discover my roots. I was told that I had an older brother, named Gilbert George Blackwood (nicknamed Noel), who lived in Jamaica, as well as an older sister named Mena Campbell (her married name) who lived in New York City. I could not wait to see my brother first, since he was out of state and living in Jamaica. In the summer of 1984, when I was thirty-two years old, I decided to take a trip to Jamaica. My daughter, Christine, my daughter's godmother, Aunt Abie, and I stayed with my deceased father's sister-in-law, Aunt Chris. Aunt Chris shared as much information as she could with me, since she was married to my father's brother. It had been so many years since I had last seen her. She used to live in New York City, but my father's brother wanted to retire in Jamaica.

When we arrived in Kingston, Jamaica, it was very, very, VERY hot! I knew my health would be okay because I was on Prednisone. My face at that time was round and puffy, but no one noticed because they had never met me, or even seen me before. When we arrived at my aunt's big house, I was scared. I did not expect to be greeted by her five dogs. We had to get used to being around the dogs because wherever my aunt was, so were the dogs.

When we all got settled we were able to meet some of the family. We did a lot of sightseeing. We visited Hope Gardens. We went to the movies and saw "Beat Street." We shopped at "Half Way Tree." We were so surprised to see that goats just walk around in the streets. Every morning, we did not have to worry about getting up because my aunt's roosters would wake us. When it was time to meet my brother for the very first time, we had to ride out to the country where he lived. When we arrived, my brother hugged me, kissed me, and then he cried. He said that he longed for this day. He also said, "Nothing happens before the time." After that, Noel asked to look at my hands. I showed them to him and he told me that I had my father's hands. I just looked down at them and smiled. After that, Noel shared so much about his life growing up with our father. I made sure to put everything he told me on tape. That way, I would always be able to hear his voice and have those beautiful memories of him.

My brother was very handy and so knowledgeable about construction work. He had built his own house from the ground up. He also showed me where he was going to put a bathroom in the house, rather than every-one having to use the outhouse.

Christine and I met so many family members and friends for the very first time. We saw so much and learned a great deal about my history. We had to make sure that we got back to Aunt Chris's house before sunset because there were no lights where my brother lived. He said that if we got stuck and were not able to leave in time, we would only be able to see via moonlight. We made sure that we hurried and returned back to my aunt's house. When we arrived, Aunt Chris and I spent some quiet time talking on the veranda about the many illnesses my dad had that he kept quiet.

Even she was not aware of how sick he was. Aunt Chris also talked about the old times when she lived in New York.

Before it was time to head back to the States, we made sure that we visited Montego Bay. It had been a very long three-week vacation and I will cherish those memories forever.

Time to Look for a New Residence

When the New Year was upon us again, I was ready to move out of the private house where my daughter and I were staying. My daughter was like my little buddy, and I would take her everywhere. She was very reserved and quiet, but also an outgoing child. I wanted nothing more than for Christine to be in an environment where there were children her own age. As I continued looking, I was able to purchase a cooperative apartment in a very nice build-ing in the Bronx. On April 1, 1985, my daughter and I moved into our new residence. It was a new beginning for the two of us and I knew we were going to love it there! I continued to take beautiful trips with my daughter when I received vacation time away from my job. That was something I always looked forward to and enjoyed.

Enrolling Christine into Mind-Builders Creative Arts Center

As soon as we got settled, I immediately registered Christine into Mind-Builders Creative Arts Center on Saturdays—where she took ballet, modern jazz and tap. She was so happy and excited to be attending.

Pursuing What I Love

During the spring of 1985, I decided to go back to school and further my education. I wanted to pursue a career in real estate. Therefore, I took some evening courses. I had been on the job for a good while and was ready to move into a totally different direction in my life.

After a little time had passed, I completed the courses and prepared myself for the exam. I passed! On November 1, 1985, I became a licensed real estate agent. I considered that to be a huge accomplishment.

Part-Time Job in the Evenings

Meanwhile, after working my full-time job during the day, I took on a real estate part-time job in the evenings. That part-time job was very convenient for me because it was directly across the street from where I was living.

Meeting My Half Sister at My Parent's House on 2/8/86

Since I had already met my half brother in Jamaica, it

was time to meet my older half sister, Mena. Mena and her two daughters, (Iva and her husband, Anthony, and her youngest daughter, Carol) were invited to my parent's house where we all met for the very first time.

We had such a nice time getting acquainted with each other and genuinely enjoyed spending the day with Mena and her family. We took so many pictures of that special day.

Taking a Trip to Walt Disney World, Orlando, Florida

On July 21, 1987 I decided to take a trip to Walt Disney World in Orlando, Florida with my daughter. I knew that was something she would definitely enjoy.

When we arrived the first day, we visited Epcot Center's 15th birthday celebration. We saw different species of tropical fish, mammals, sharks, dolphins, etc. We took a cruise that takes you through the tropical rain forest, African desert, and the Magic Kingdom. The Disney characters put on a very nice show, and we took lots of pictures with them. At the end of the night, there was a beautiful electronic circus. We also went to the sea aquarium and fantasy theatre, which included a magic show. We saw a 'home of the future', called Xanadu. The house had a talking computer that you had to challenge. Christine really had fun with that.

We had a great, exciting, and fun trip together. We returned home on Monday, July 27, 1987.

Part-Time Job Comes to a Close

After working my real estate part-time job for two years, and getting the experience I needed, on October 31, 1987 I was able to stop working that job. I realized that I wanted to pursue a more active role as a legal secretary for a real estate company.

Letter from Child Support

I received a letter from the court on May 13, 1988 stating that my ex-husband was in arrears; I had not been receiving child support payments as was ordered. My records were updated so that child support enforcement activity could be continued on my behalf. I had to fill out the form they sent me so that I could receive the support to which my daughter was entitled.

Seeking a New Position

One morning, I was quietly sitting at home and looking through the January 22, 1989 newspaper. I wanted to see what jobs were out there that I might be interested in. I came across an ad that just fit me perfectly. It was a position for a legal secretary to work with a leading real estate management company. It required the knowledge of Multi-Mate, which was a word processing computer skill. That was good to see because I already had experience using Multi-Mate. They needed someone who had commercial leasing or real estate experience to work in their legal department. Plus, they were willing to train the right person. They were offering good benefits, vacation, and an excellent starting salary. I was too happy when I saw that ad because I already had all the skills they needed. I did not waste any time and called the company first thing that Monday morning. An appointment was set for me to meet with them that coming Friday.

When I arrived at the interview, what took me by surprise was the well-received atmosphere of the company. Bob, who was the one looking for a legal secretary, started looking over my resume. He was very impressed because he saw that I used the same word processing skill that they used. Plus, I had many years of legal experience. To top it all off, I had my real estate license. Next, he wanted to dictate a letter to me. He said that he was looking for correct spelling, grammar, punctuation, and neatness. He wanted the letter to be done in whatever shorthand style I used.

After the test was administered, Bob took the letter I had typed, along with my shorthand notes. I proceeded back to his office. He informed me that my letter was perfect, as well as my computer and shorthand skills. I was hired on the spot. I had a great weekend after receiving such good news!

Breaking the News to My Job

After thirteen years of service, I had to break the news to my job that I would be officially leaving the company. I informed Mrs. Klein, who was my boss, that I had been offered a position with one of the top leading real estate companies in Midtown Manhattan and that I would be leaving in a week. They were all shocked, surprised, happy, and hurt. I told Mrs. Klein that the real estate company made me an offer that I could not refuse. She tried so hard to see if they could possibly offer me more money to stay, but to her surprise, they could not compete with the high salary the new job was willing to give me. Therefore, it was time for me to move on. I was issued a beautiful letter of recommendation.

My sendoff by The General Contractors Association was a beautiful one! I had grown and learned so much from working with the GCA team. It was an honor and a privilege to have worked with such a great company as that.

I was also grateful to have bosses that thought so highly of me, that they were willing to handle my divorce and child support proceedings during that very important time in my life.

Employed by One of the Top Leading Real Estate Owner/Developer Management Companies in Manhattan

It was Ash Wednesday on February 8, 1989, and I had just started working with the new real estate company. I was willing and ready to learn about the residential and commercial side of real estate, which had always been a passion of mine.

After getting completely adjusted to working with the company in their Midtown office, they decided that—due to their continuing growth and expansion—

they were ready to move to a new location. They were moving their main office to downtown New Rochelle. The owners of the company had started asking the employees whether or not we would like to work at their new location. That was an excellent choice for me. The bus stop near my home was the first stop and it would take me straight downtown to New Rochelle. I was glad because I knew that I would be able to always get a seat.

The day that I actually saw our new office building for the very first time was wonderful; it was just beautiful. It felt so good to be working in a brand new environment with such a great company.

What I Did to Myself at Age Thirty-Seven

One day, when I was thirty-seven years old, I tried to move my very long, heavy dresser from one side of the bedroom to the other. I would usually take out all of the dresser drawers first, before even attempting to move it; but unfortunately, on February 5, 1990, I did not do that. As I proceeded to push my dresser across the red carpet floor, all of a sudden, I could feel a tear—like something had just ripped open inside of me. I immediately stopped. I bent down to touch my stomach just a little below my navel. There was a little soft pocket sticking out; so, I gently pushed it back in, but then I had to do it again. It just kept popping back out. I said to myself, *Oh no, something bad has happened.* I started having pain and knew that I needed to get to the hospital. I could not believe what I did to myself.

I went to the Jack D. Weiler Hospital at the Albert

Einstein College of Medicine. The diagnosis was a right inguinal hernia. The symptoms were pain and a lump to the right of my groin. Findings determined that I had a right groin hernia.

I was hospitalized on February 6, 1990, and the right inguinal hernia repair was done right away. The doctor did an excellent job. I was discharged on February 7, 1990. After coming home, I was in so much pain. It was very hard for me to walk or even stand up straight.

I informed my boss that I would probably be coming back to work in March. I was slowly, but surely starting to feel pretty good again. On March 14, 1990, I was examined by my doctor, and I had a very good report. He said that it was definitely okay for me to return back to work first thing that next morning.

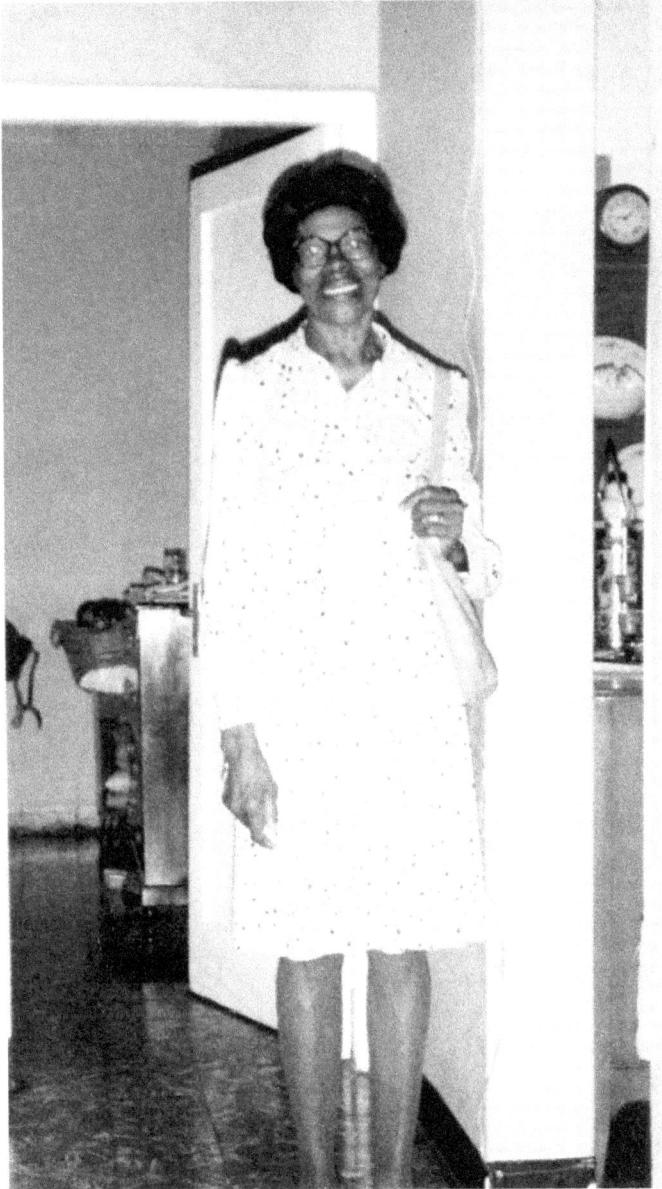

My Aunt Chris at her home in Kingston, Jamaica
Summer of 1984. She was on her way to run errands.

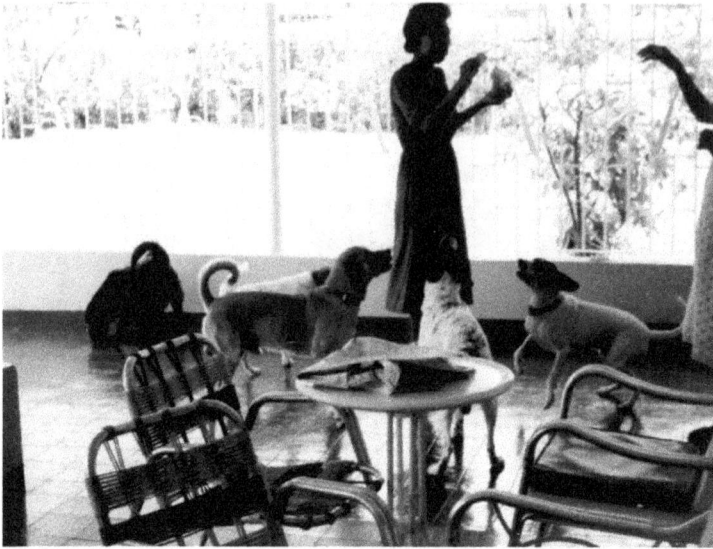

A friend visiting my Aunt. Aunt Chris had five very nice dogs - Summer of 1984.

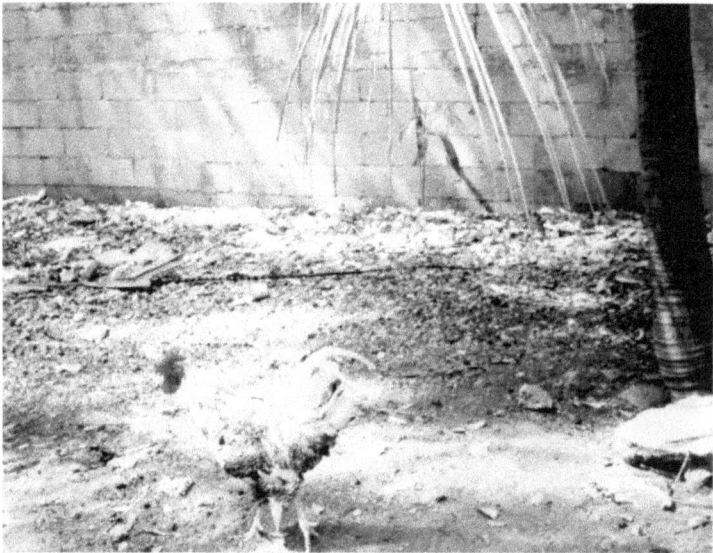

This was one of the roosters who woke us up every morning - Summer of 1984.

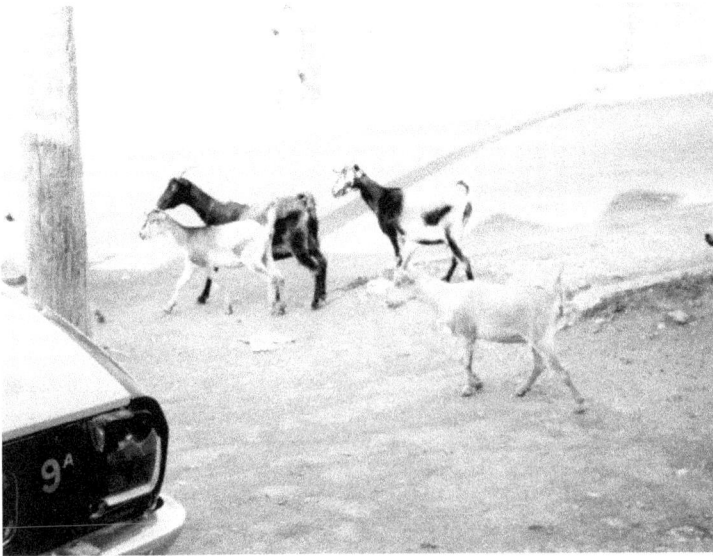

The goats roam around the streets - Summer of 1984.

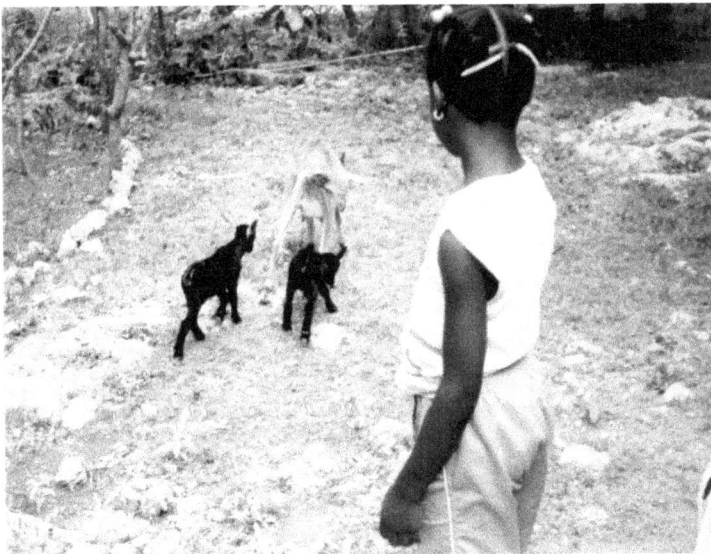

My daughter, Christine amazed at the goats - Summer of 1984.

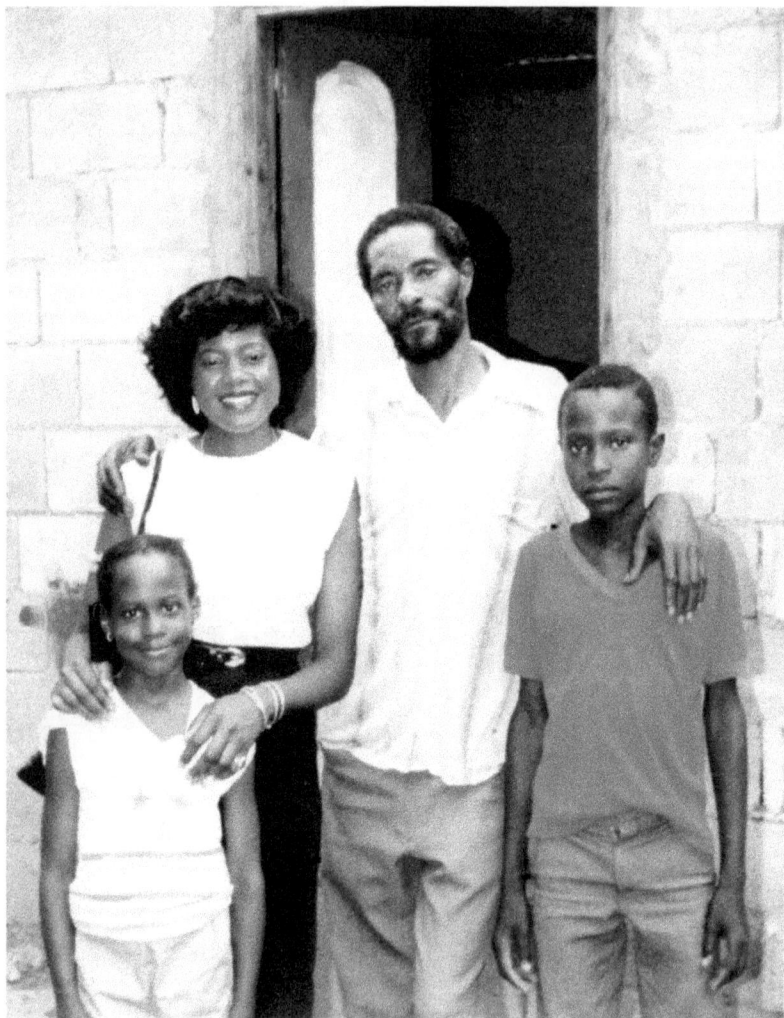

In Clarendon - Summer of 1984. My daughter and I meeting my half brother, Gilbert Blackwood, and his young son for the very first time.

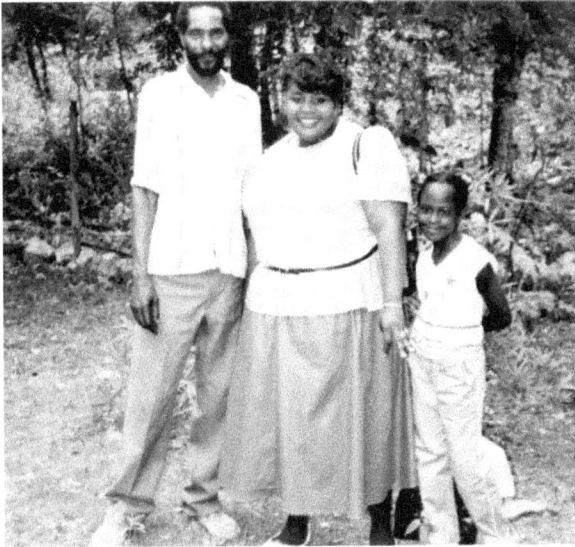

Left to right: My half brother, Gilbert, my daughter's godmother, Aunt Abie, and my daughter, Christine - Summer of 1984.

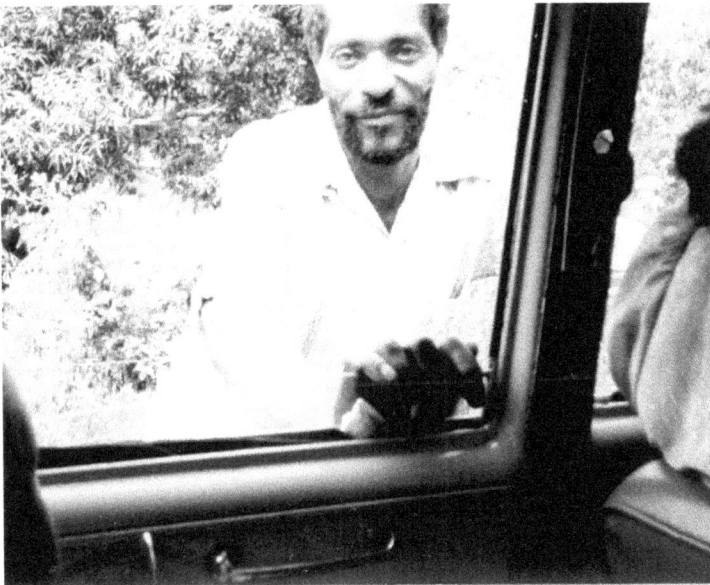

My brother, Gilbert looking on as we were headed back to my Aunt's house - Summer of 1984.

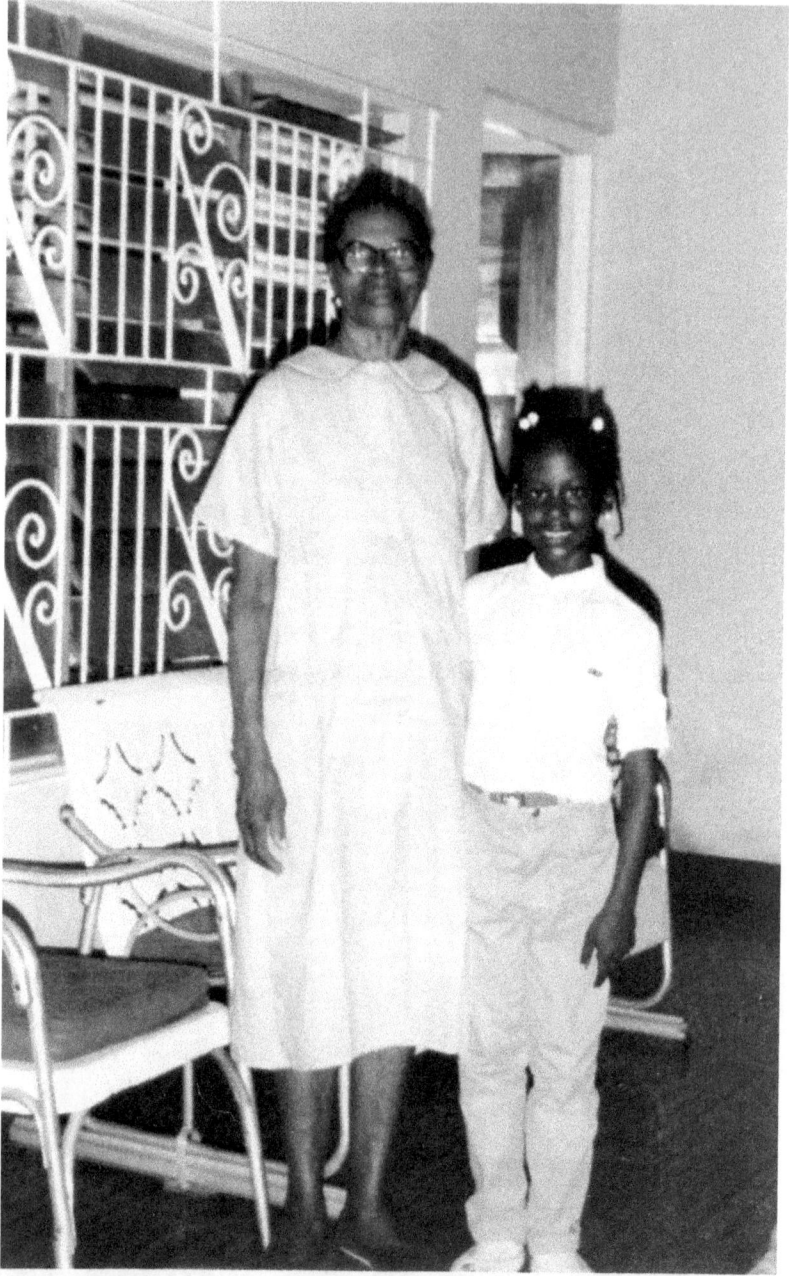

My Aunt Chris, and my daughter, Christine on the veranda
Summer of 1984.

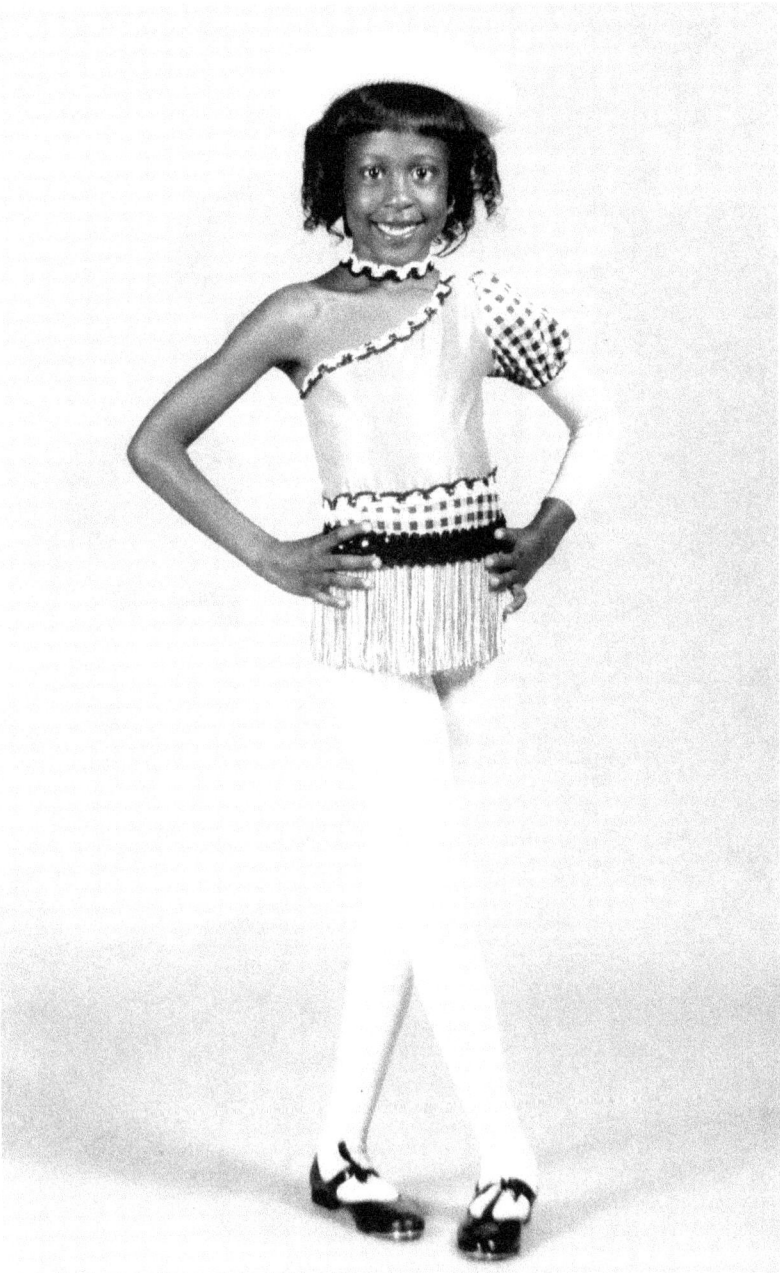

Christine enrolled in Mind-Builders Creative Arts Center.
She was seven years old.

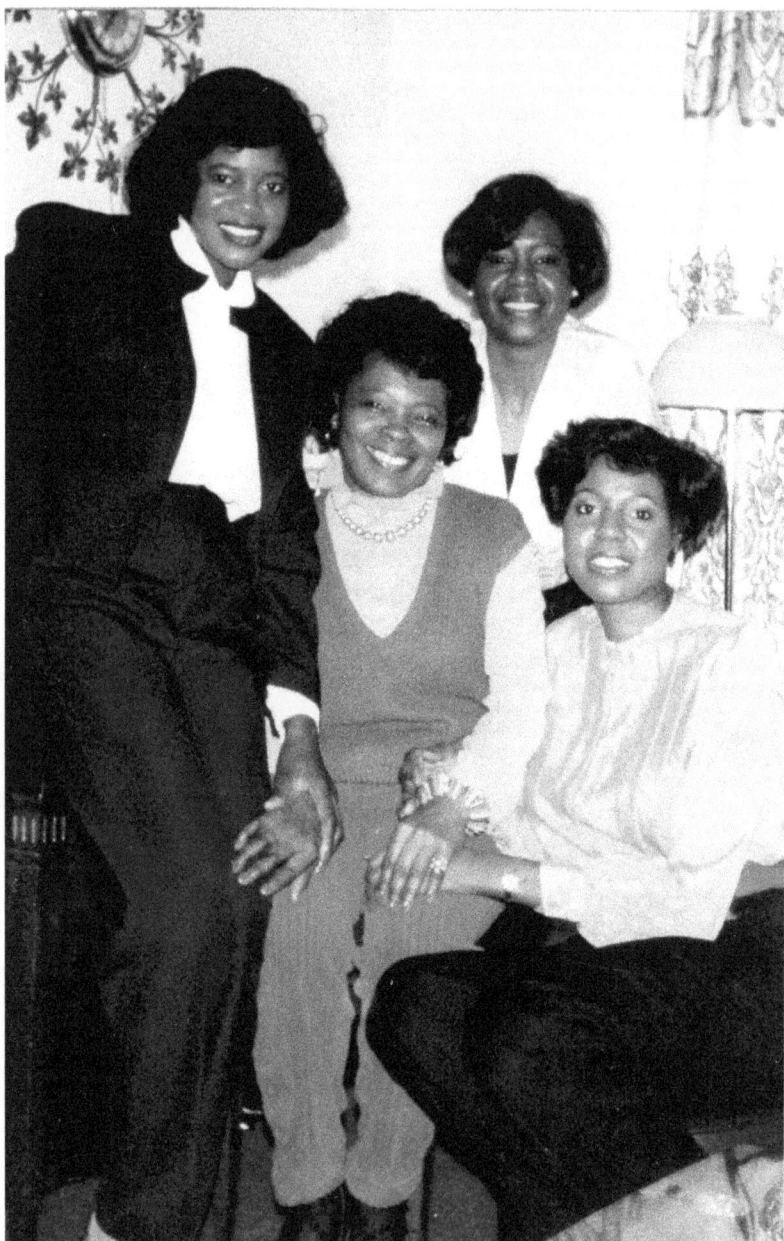

Meeting my half sister, Mena for the very first time - February 8, 1986. Top back: My sister, Vanessa. Left to right: Me, Mena, and Claudette.

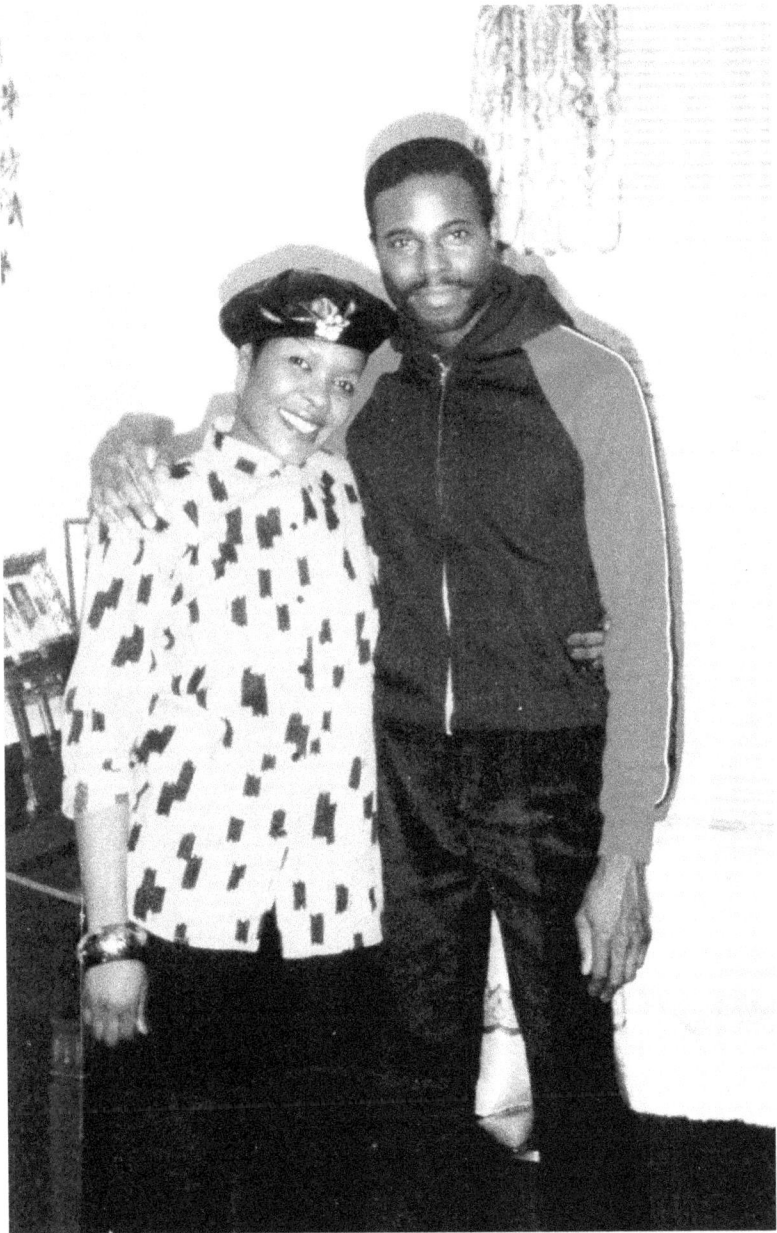

Mena's daughter, Iva and my brother, Reginald - February 8, 1986.

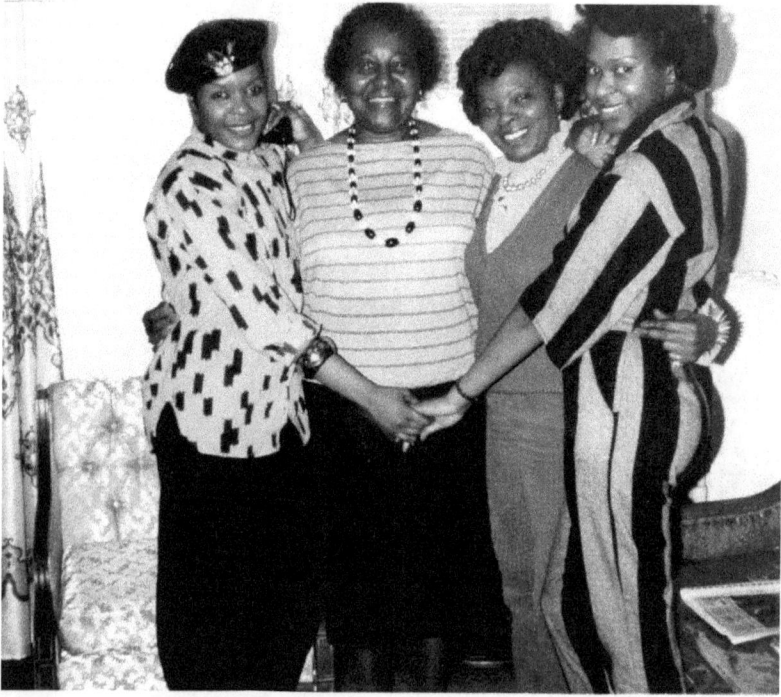

Left to right: Mena's daughter Iva, my mother, Mena, Mena's daughter, Carol - February 8, 1986.

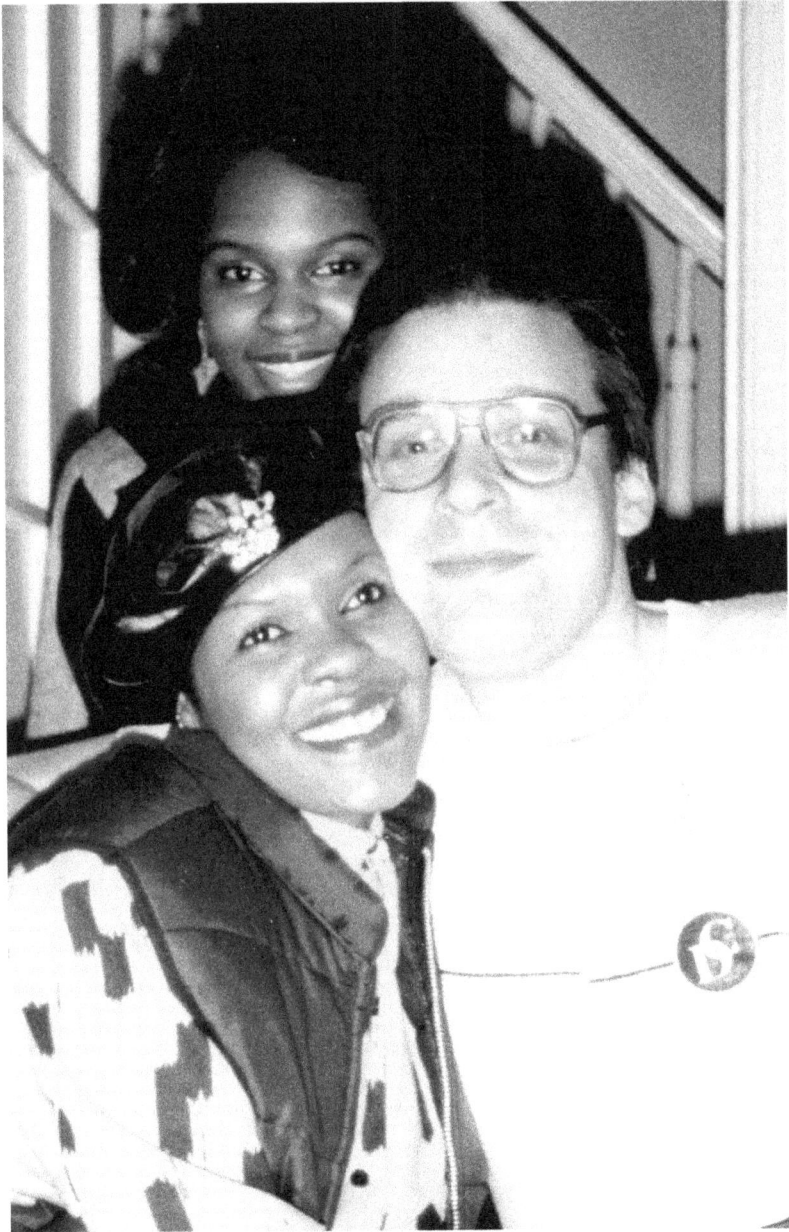

Top: Carol
Bottom: Iva and her husband Anthony - February 8, 1986.

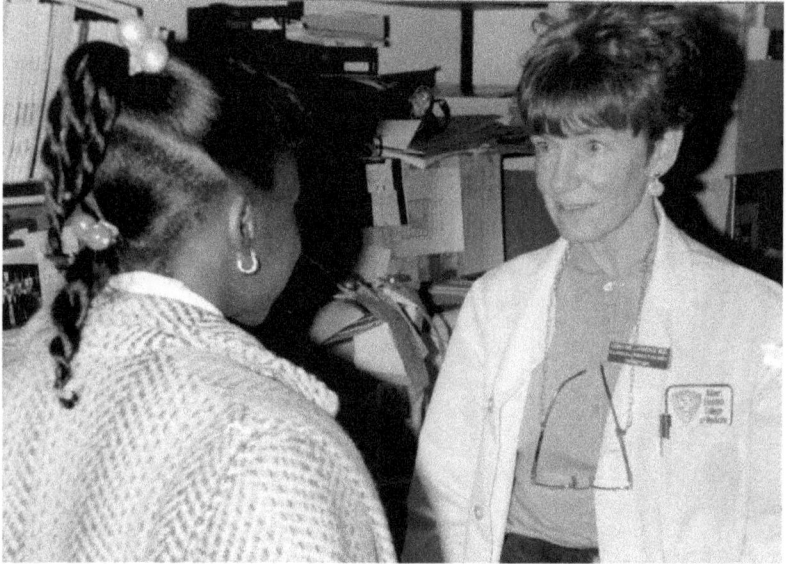

My daughter, Christine visiting with Dr. Christine Lawrence.

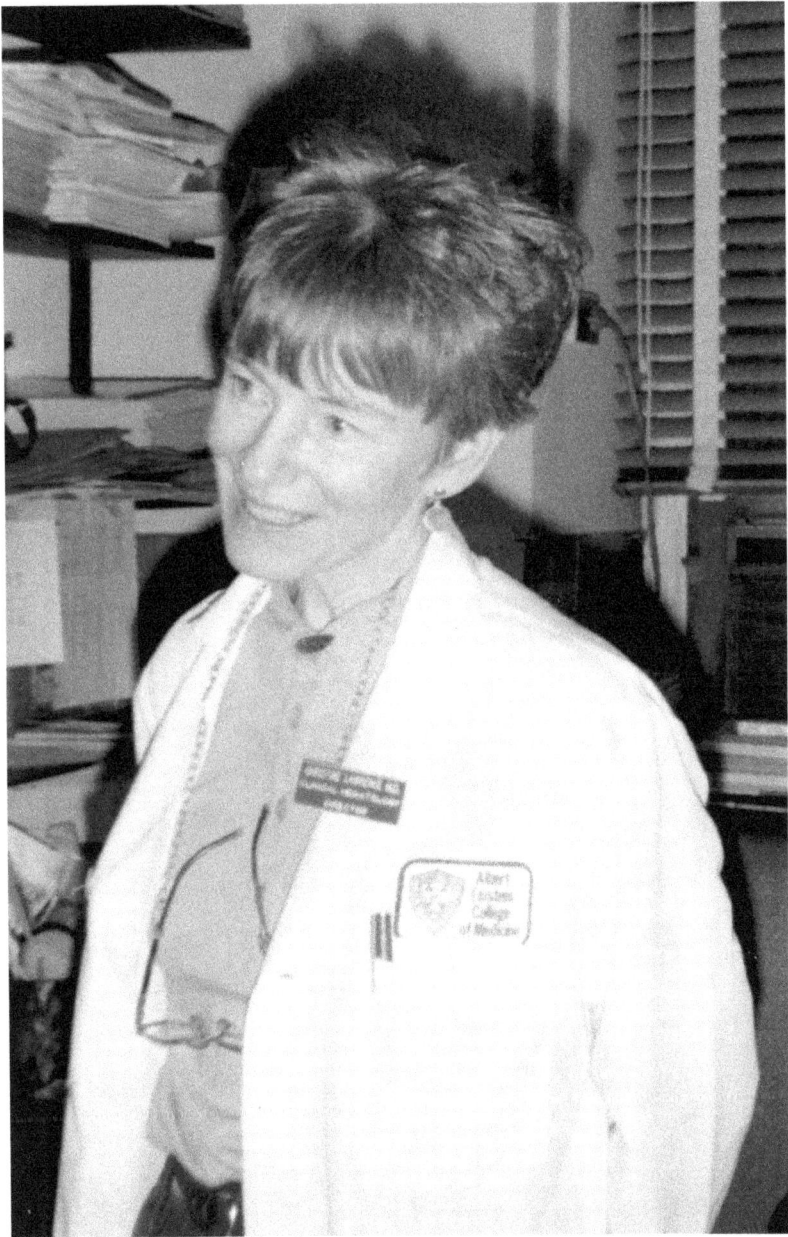

Dr. Christine Lawrence speaking with my daughter, Christine.

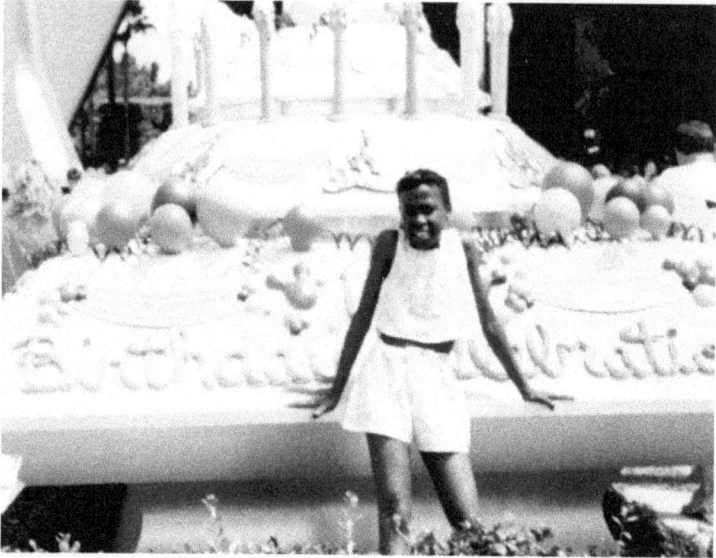

My daughter, Christine at Epcot's 15th birthday celebration in Orlando, Florida - July 1987.

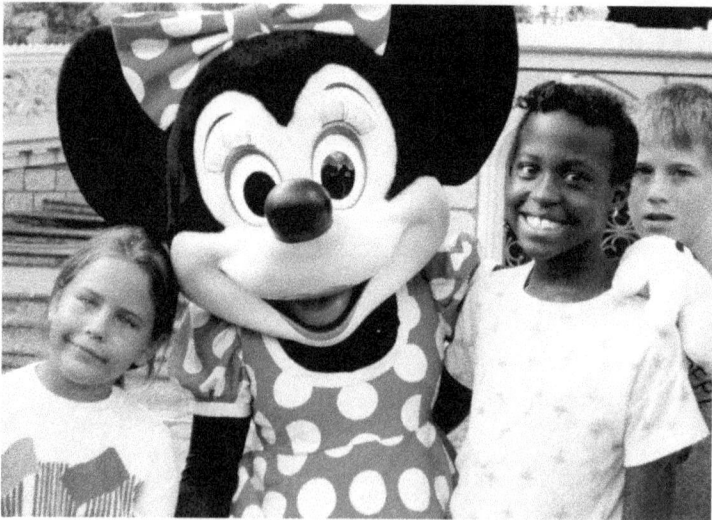

My daughter, Christine, and Minnie Mouse - July 1987.

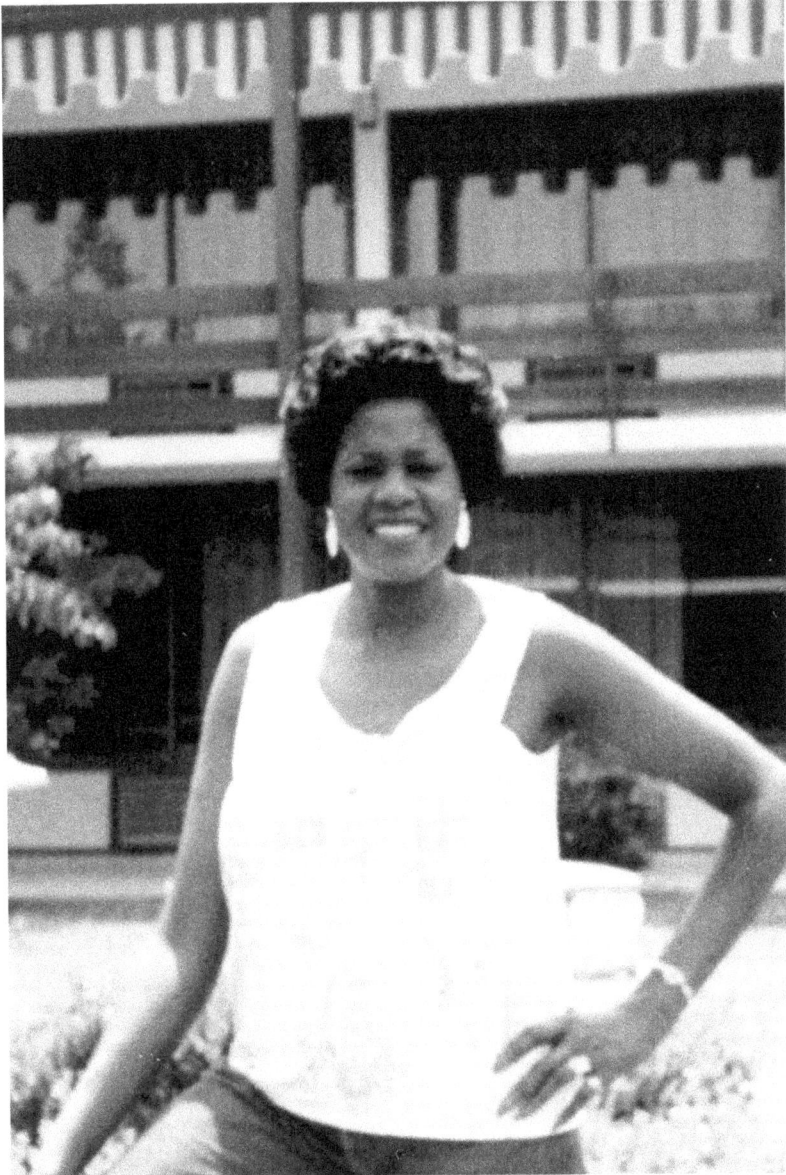

Across from the hotel where my daughter and I were staying - July 1987.

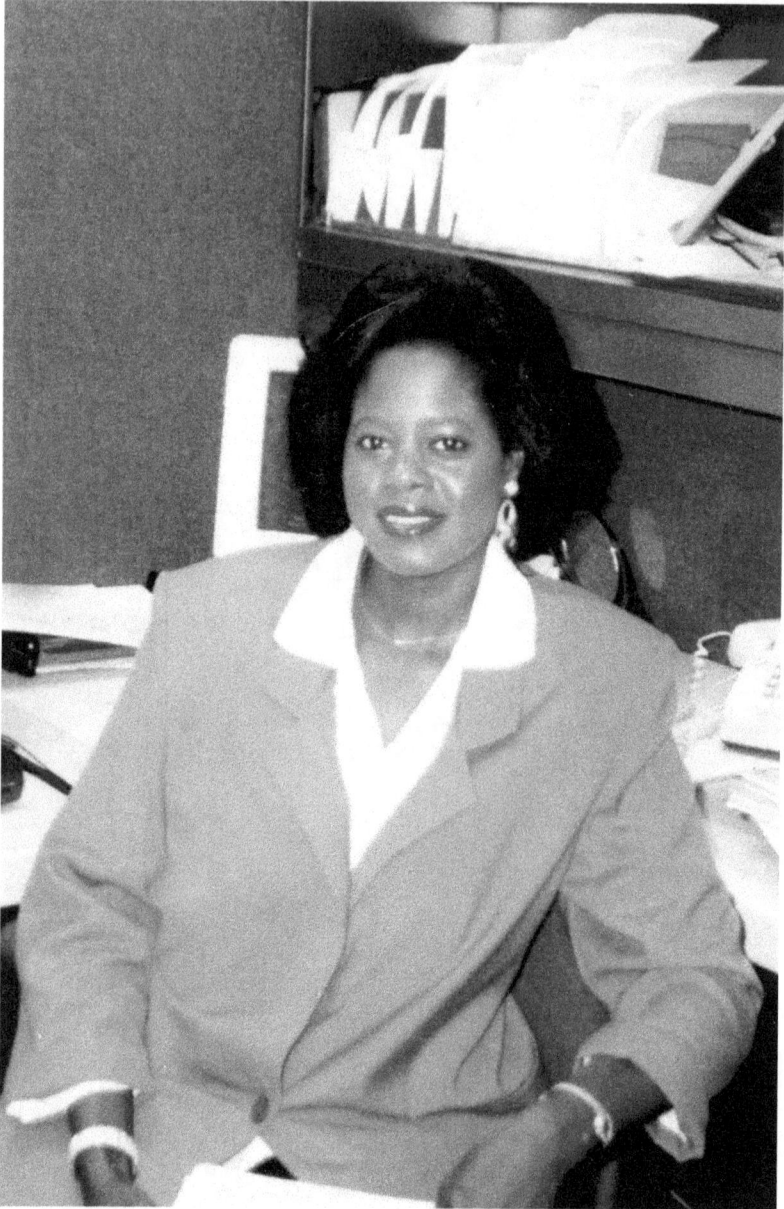

Working for a family-owned real estate company in New York City during 1989.

CHAPTER 5

LIFE AFTER OPERATION

I really enjoyed going to work from the Bronx to New Rochelle, especially with the bus stop being down the street from where I lived. I loved being able to sit by the window in the morning. When the bus stopped in Mount Vernon, it started getting pretty crowded. There was a guy who always made it a point to smile and say hello every time he saw me—before he proceeded to the back of the bus. He also knew that, when my stop came, I always got off at the back entrance of the bus. As my stop approached, I could feel him staring me down until the back door opened and I got off.

That had been going on for at least five months or longer. One day, it was a holiday and the bus was no longer crowded, that same guy asked me, "Is it okay if I sit here?" I nodded 'yes' and we started talking—phone numbers were exchanged, and after that, we started dating. It wasn't long before we decided that we were ready for a more exclusive relationship. His name was

Melvin.

Ready to Have a Child

When I was thirty-eight years old, I felt that it was time for me to have a child. I had always said that my cutoff time for having a child was forty. Melvin and I had decided that we were both ready to have a child. So, I was very happy when I became pregnant. Dr. Samuel Oberlander, who delivered my first child fourteen years prior, would also be overseeing my second pregnancy. How beautiful was that!

Amniocentesis Done – 9/18/90

Melvin had been constantly telling me, over and over again, that we were having a boy. So, on September 18, 1990, when my fetus was just a little over four months developed, I had an Amniocentesis done at the Kennedy Center in New York City. At that time, I was able to find out the sex of the baby. Melvin had predicted right. We were having a boy! We were both very excited.

Lamaze Classes

After hearing the good news about my baby, I wanted to make sure that I would be better prepared having my second child. The entire nine months being pregnant with my first child was excellent, but the delivery was challenging. I was scared, did not know what to expect, and was inexperienced. I did not want to make the same mistake twice. Therefore, Melvin and I had started taking Lamaze classes together.

After all of our classes were over, on January 28, 1991, Melvin and I received a document certifying that we both completed a course in Psychoprophylactic Preparation for Childbirth. During that eight month of my pregnancy, I was so glad to have accomplished that. I looked forward to an easy delivery.

I Was in Labor

Oh no! It was Monday, February 18, 1991, and I had started to have contractions. We immediately went to the Albert Einstein/Weiler Hospital in the Bronx, New York. While we were at the hospital, Dr. Oberlander informed my family that they did not have to leave my bedside. He told them that if they would like to, they could stay right there with me in the same room and see the delivery of my little boy. My daughter, Melvin, and my parents were all there for the birth of my baby. But, my mother was the only one who wanted to stay in the room with me to see the delivery.

As Dr. Oberlander started examining me, he said that the baby's cord seemed to be wrapped around a part of the baby's body and it was very hard for him to determine where. It had been a total of eight hours. Dr. Oberlander had to induce me. When it was time for the birth of my baby, I began pushing and the baby started to come out. I could see the expression on my mother's face. It looked like she wanted to throw up.

My Baby Was Born

My little baby boy was born at 3:44 AM. He weighed 6 lbs. 6½ oz. and was 19½ inches long. He also had his father's blood type. I named him Christopher because that was the first name that continued to follow from my first doctor, named Christine. My baby's middle name was Samuel, named after my OB/GYN who delivered him. Therefore, my little boy's full name is Christopher Samuel Bethune. That was an excellent name for him and it seemed to fit him perfectly! After everything was all over my mother said, that was such an experience to see and one that she would never forget.

My hospital stay was a beautiful one! The day before I could leave with my little boy, the hospital surprised us with a very special dinner that was set up beautifully for us. On February 20, 1991, I was discharged. I had two beautiful children, Christine and Christopher, in my life to take care of.

Christopher's Baby Shower and Christening Day (All in One)

On March 16, 1991, we celebrated my son, Christopher Samuel Bethune's, beautiful day! His baby shower was being held at my parent's house. That morning, we all headed to my son's Christening, which was being held at Crawford Memorial United Methodist Church in the Bronx, New York. Immediately after, everyone returned back to my parent's house for the rest of the evening. Many family and friends were there to celebrate that special occasion of ours. We had a very big turnout!

After I received my six-week thorough checkup, my doctor said that everything was fine. I returned back to work during the month of April, 1991.

Christine Continued Her Craft

Christine was still attending Mind-Builders Creative Arts Center. She learned a great deal and continued to receive plenty of awards for all of her performances. She also enjoyed when I would take her to see different theatre performances. She was always so enthused when the narrator would start speaking. That always got her attention, and I knew there was something there. She was always the type of person that needed to stay active.

Lupus Flare-up – 7/2/91

I had a clinic appointment to see Dr. Diamond on July 2, 1991, and my ankles were very badly swollen. Dr. Diamond said that I was having a lupus flare-up. She started me on three 5 mg Prednisone pills a day, three Iron pills a day, one Potassium pill, one Hydrochlorothiazide pill, and one multi-vitamin/mineral supplement. My weight was 175 pounds. I would have really liked to have taken off those thirty extra pounds that I had gained from my pregnancy with my son before getting back on Prednisone.

My Stepbrother's Passing – 8/13/91

On August 6, 1991, my stepbrother Major Colley, Jr. (named after his father) was admitted into Harlem Hospital. My father knew that his forty-one-year-old son was headed down the wrong path in his life because of his drug usage. On August 13, 1991, at 9:55 AM, he passed away at Harlem Hospital. For so long, my stepfather tried to encourage Junior (the name we called my stepbrother) to do the right thing, but the street life got the best of him. My stepbrother's death took a toll on my father and he was not the same after that.

A Poem to Her Grandmother

When my daughter, Christine, was thirteen and a half years old—and already very talented in many areas of her young life—we were looking through the *Kids Today* newspaper. They were asking children to send in poems that they had written. They said, "You must include your name, birthday, city and state. If selected, it will be published in the *Kids Today* newspaper." I knew that Christine would definitely like to do that.

A little time had passed after Christine sent in her poem. I had not been buying the newspaper on a regular basis. So, on Sunday, September 15, 1991, I decided to pick up *The New York Times,* as well as the *Kids Today* newspaper. After getting myself comfortable at home and looking through both newspapers, I came across a poem that read:

Lil' ol' Grandma Colley sang herself to sleep.
She had her 40 winks, and her dreams she'd be
    sure to keep.
In the morning she got herself away from her
    lil' ol' tiny bed.
"I didn't want to sleep all day!" Lil' ol' Grandma
    Colley said.
Lil' ol' Grandma Colley strutted herself to the
    kitchen.
'Cause there would be a whole bowl of pancakes
    she had to be mixin.'
After she ate breakfast she went out for some air.
Even though it was cold outside, she didn't
    really care.
When she came in, she felt like drinking some
    hot herbal tea.
But when she found no tea bags, she said, "Oh
    no, this couldn't be!"
Later on Lil' ol' Grandma Colley decided to
    get away.
Lil' ol' Grandma Colley sang herself to sleep.
She had to get her 40 winks, and her dreams
    she'd be sure to keep.

Christine Horn   Age 13½
Bronx, N.Y.

I immediately called out to Christine and told her
to come see her poetry in the *Kids Today* newspaper. We
could not believe that they did not even let us know that
her poem was selected. If I had not decided to pick up the

newspaper on Sunday, I would have never even known that my daughter's poem was published. I congratulated my daughter for doing such an excellent job submitting her poetry and for acknowledging her grandmother, Mrs. Lillian Colley, my mother.

I Was Pregnant

We were in the New Year of 1992, when I noticed that I was feeling a little different. It was something that I could not even explain. I had just found out that I was pregnant. I had always said that forty was my cutoff age for having a child. At that time, I was thirty-nine years old.

I was also running out of space in my nice cooperative apartment. I had to decide quickly on what to do, since I was having my third child. I asked myself, *Should I get a bigger cooperative apartment in this development? Or, do I want to look for a house of my own?* That was something I needed to consider.

My first priority was definitely my young teenage daughter. She had so much talent inside of her that just needed to be explored. Christine always said to me, "Mommy, do you want to stay in New York City all of your life?" I would just look at her. But, before I would even give her an answer, she would immediately say to me, "Not me! When I get older, I won't be living here all of my life. I'll be moving somewhere else." I think hearing my daughter say that gave me the answer I was searching for.

Ever since Christine was a little girl, she would always tell me – in no specific order – that she wanted to become an actress, a dancer, a singer, and a model. Her goals have never changed. With the many talents that I knew she had, she might go unnoticed living in New York. New York City is such a big place, that I really needed to explore other options for her. As much as it was definitely going to be a great big sacrifice for me, I had to do what I felt was best. Therefore, I took it upon myself and started looking at different places in New York City in which to live. When my mother was available, I would also take her with me. I was not at all happy with the places that I was seeing and knew that something had to change.

Time to Take a Trip

At the beginning of 1992, I felt that it was time for my daughter and I to take a trip. Since Christine would be out of school for the Easter holiday, I thought that would be a great time for us to take a trip to Atlanta, Georgia. I heard that Atlanta was known for the arts and knew that was something my daughter would really love. I also felt that she needed to be surrounded by people her own age, doing positive things.

So, to better prepare for that trip, I contacted two brokers that I would be able to see, as well as a school that I was interested in visiting. That way, when we arrived, I would know how to balance my schedule. My ex-husband's sister, Nancy, told me that her cousin, Jean, also lived in Georgia, and that I should contact her. So, I did.

We had a good flight. Christine was amazed by how beautiful Atlanta looked. The first thing that I asked her when we got off the airplane was whether she thought she could live in Atlanta. She said, "Sure!" At that very moment, that was all I needed to hear. We were staying at the Days Inn in Decatur, Georgia, which was not too far from Nancy's cousin. Jean was so nice to show us around. I also told my daughter that we would be looking at some houses. Christine was so used to me looking at houses, that she thought we were just sightseeing as usual.

I had one broker who took us around in the morning hours and the other broker took us around in the evenings. I continued to keep moving forward. With all that was happening so fast, Christine was also encouraging her little brother to walk. After a few days, Christine had him walking! That was such a big relief for us, especially since I was a few months pregnant.

After a short time had passed from looking at houses, we finally found a house that we liked. It was in the same district as the school that I had already contacted before leaving New York. It was called Tri-Cities High School (Performing Arts School). After taking a tour of the school, Christine was so excited. We were told that Christine would need to audition, but once they saw her outstanding grades, they said that she would not have to audition after all. Christine ended up being accepted into Tri-Cities High School when school resumed in August.

Christine still had no idea that we would be relocating to Atlanta, Georgia. She thought that we were just in Atlanta having a wonderful, beautiful Easter break vacation. I also enjoyed seeing Jean. She was so kind to welcome us to her home so that we would be able to share a very special Easter Sunday dinner with her family. That was so nice of her to do that.

Our time was over, after having a wonderful time in Georgia. When we arrived back in New York, I ended up closing on the house that we found. It was going to be done by mail, which was good for me. The couple that I bought the house from was not ready to move out until the end of June. That timing was perfect for me, since Christine would be out of school. Therefore, I asked them if it would be okay for the broker to take some pictures of the house to send to me. They said that was fine.

I could not believe from all the excitement that we had on our nice vacation in Georgia, that Christine still had no idea that we were moving. She never even questioned me about our relocating. So, I did not say anything.

In private, I began telling Melvin that we found a house in Georgia. He was surprised. I told him that we would be moving to Atlanta the same day that Christine gets out of school. He was happy because he was ready for a change as well. Since, I was pregnant and would not be able to work, Melvin would have to find a job when we got there. He has always been good about letting me handle his money.

In the meantime, I was glad that my broker sent me pictures of the house. She informed me that it took so many rolls of film just to get a decent set of pictures. I thanked her for the effort. I appreciated her doing that for me. As I was carefully looking through the pictures, I noticed that there was a bible in each of the bedrooms. I was a little surprised, so I quickly called the broker and asked her to contact the owners to find out why there were bibles in the bedrooms. The wife told my broker that this was always something her grandmother told her to do. She said that the bible would give the house a positive feel.

News to Tell My Job and My Ex-husband

I had to break the news to my job and my ex-husband that I would be moving out of state and relocating to Atlanta, Georgia in June.

I was going to miss my job very much because I really loved what I was doing, but I felt that I had to do what I thought was best for my family and I. After discussing my move with my job, they were happy for me, but sorry to hear that I would be leaving. They had always treated me extremely well and I did well working with such a great company. My boss told me that I was going to "God's country." I did not question him about that, but was surprised to hear him say it. I did not know what the future was going to hold, but since I was pregnant with my third child, I felt the need and the sacrifice to keep moving forward.

I informed Robert that we would be moving out-of-state in June. He was shocked. He thought that moving to the South would be good for his daughter because it was not so fast-paced, like New York City is.

On May 2, 1992, I found a moving company that was located in New Jersey that would move us all the way to Atlanta, Georgia. All of the paperwork had been signed, and I was able to proceed with my move.

Amniocentesis Done – 5/12/92

Melvin had told me, over and over, that I was having a little girl this time. He would always put his ear to my stomach and say, "There's a little girl in there." Or, he would say, "There's a little Valerie in there." So, on May 12, 1992, I had an Amniocentesis done. Everything went well at the Albert Einstein College of Medicine – Montefiore Medical Center. It turned out that Melvin was right again. I was having a girl! I was happy to be sharing our good news with my daughter.

Breaking the News to My Daughter, Christine

The time was near. I had to finally break the news to my daughter that we were moving. I was ready to explain to her exactly what was really going on and what was about to happen.

Me: "Christine, remember when we went to Atlanta, Georgia?"

Christine: "Yes, Mommy."

Me: "Remember when we were looking at all the different houses and the school that you saw in Georgia?"

Christine: "Yes, Mommy."

Me: "Remember the last house that we both liked?"

Christine: "Yes, Mommy."

Me: "Well…I bought that house!"

Christine: "You bought that house?"

Me: "Yes. Remember when we got off the plane and I asked you if you could live in Georgia?"

Christine: "Yes, Mommy."

Me: "That's when I went forward and we started looking at houses."

Christine: "I knew how you always liked looking at houses, but I thought you were just doing it for fun, but not to live there!"

Me: "Remember, when you used to ask me, 'Mommy do you want to live in New York City all your life?' And, with that little smart mouth of yours, you said to me, 'Not me! When I grow up, I won't be living here all my life.'"

Christine: "Mommy, you tricked me!"

At that very moment, Christine was feeling a little hurt. She could not believe what I had done. So, to make her feel a little better, I proceeded to tell her that the Performing Arts School that she saw was in the same district as the neighborhood where we bought the house. I also told her that time would move quickly for her and maybe she would not be too bored since Georgia's schools open in August—she would not have to wait until September like the schools in New York. Plus, the summer months could give Christine an opportunity to get more acquainted with her new home. After hearing all of that, she started to feel somewhat happy about the school she would be attending.

My daughter was looking so bored during her teenage years living in New York, and I felt that something needed to change for her benefit. I told her that she had so much talent that just needed to come out. When we move to Georgia and she starts school, her life would definitely change. After she heard everything that I was saying, it started to sink in and I noticed that she was getting anxious.

She proceeded to tell me that, if we did stay in New York, she would have to take swimming classes in order to graduate out of high school. In that particular situation, Christine was glad that we were moving because she did not want to take swimming.

I told Christine that when I attended high school, I also had to take swimming or I would not have been able to graduate. I, on the other hand, had to take swimming during the winter months and I was not happy at all. Plus, the worst part of it all was that my swimming class started very early in the morning. We had to dive off the diving board and into a floating position in order to pass the class. I was happy that I was able to do it and I passed.

Christine continued to say that she was happy that we were moving and that she did not have to take swimming. She was fourteen years old and looked forward to what lies ahead for her in Georgia. I was looking forward to meeting my new doctors and to my new baby being born.

Time flew by so fast for all of us. Christine said that she still did not have enough time to tell some of her friends that she was moving out of state. I told her not to worry because things have a way of always working out somehow. On June 22, 1992, the moving company came over to my apartment and finalized everything. They took a motor vehicle descriptive inventory of my car and Melvin's car, and all of the furniture that would be going on the truck and shipped to the new address in Georgia.

It was the day before my birthday on June 26, 1992, and there was so much excitement going on. My girl-friend, Jackie, had quickly stopped by to see me before I left. I also had to clear up some last minute details with my cooperative apartment. Therefore, I missed my flight trying to make it to Atlanta, Georgia that day. I had to call the airlines to reschedule. Luckily for me, I told them that it was my birthday that following day and they did not charge me any extra fees for flying out that day.

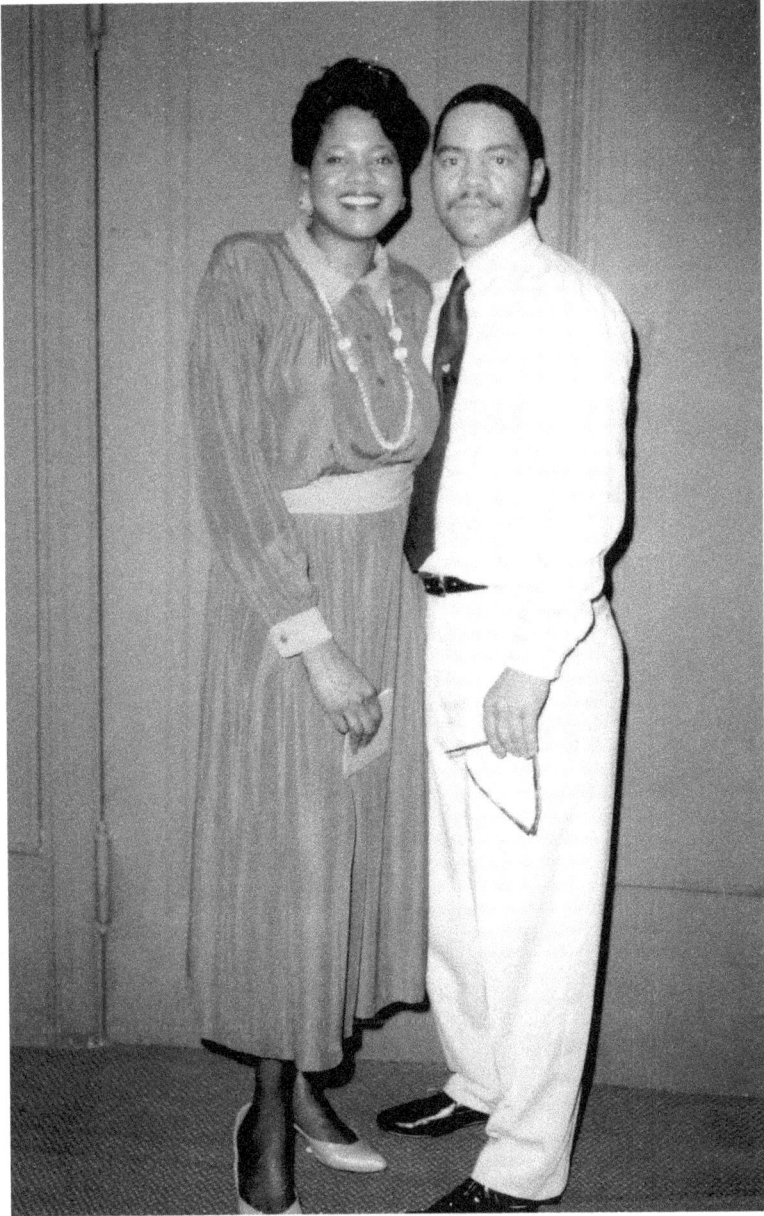

Melvin and I were at "Savage Discotheque."
May 27, 1990, in New York City.

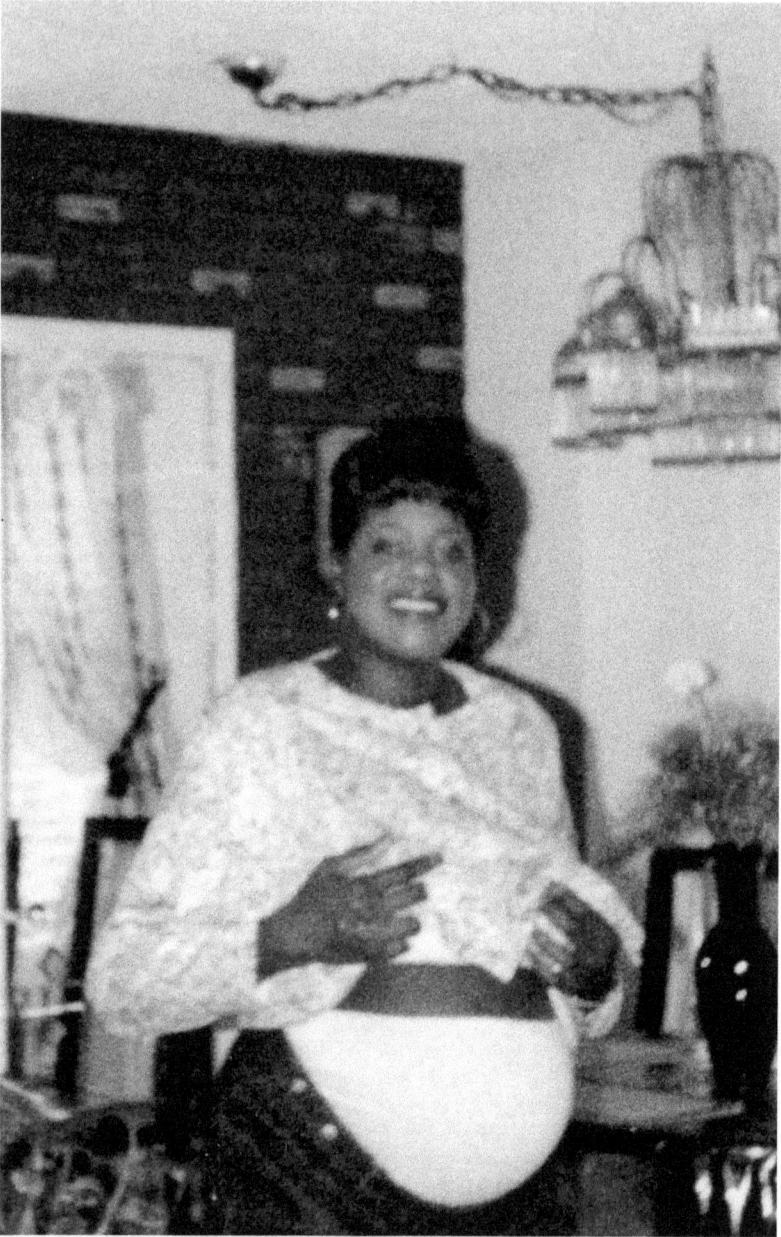

At home. I was pregnant with my baby boy.

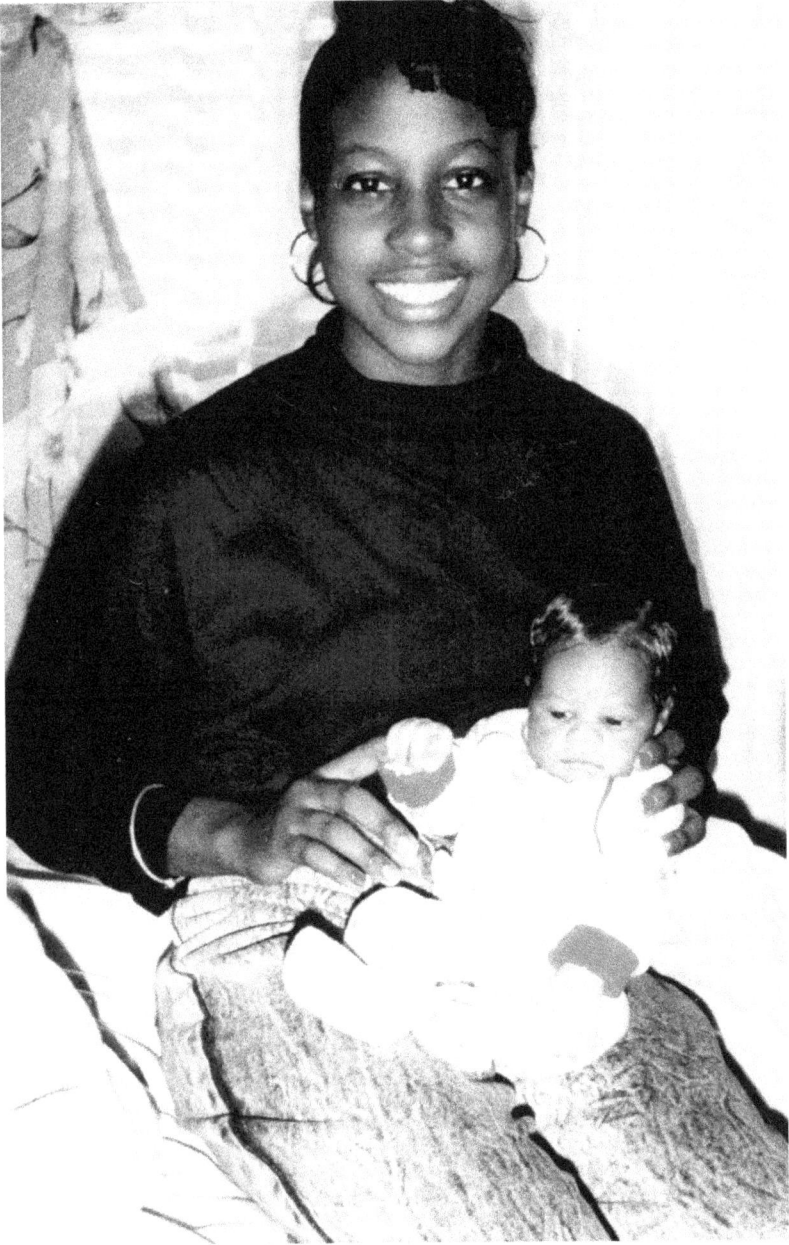

My daughter, Christine and her new brother, Christopher at home.

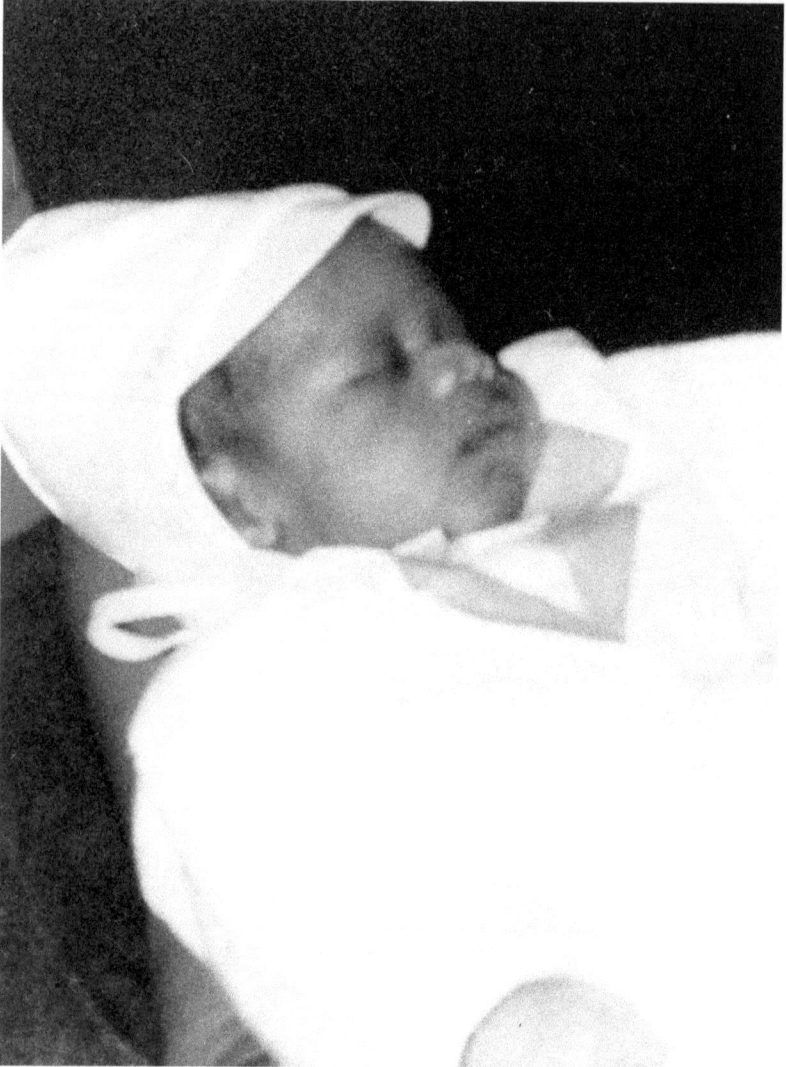

Christopher Samuel Bethune's Christening and Baby Shower
He was three and a half weeks old and sleeping through his
beautiful day - March 16, 1991.

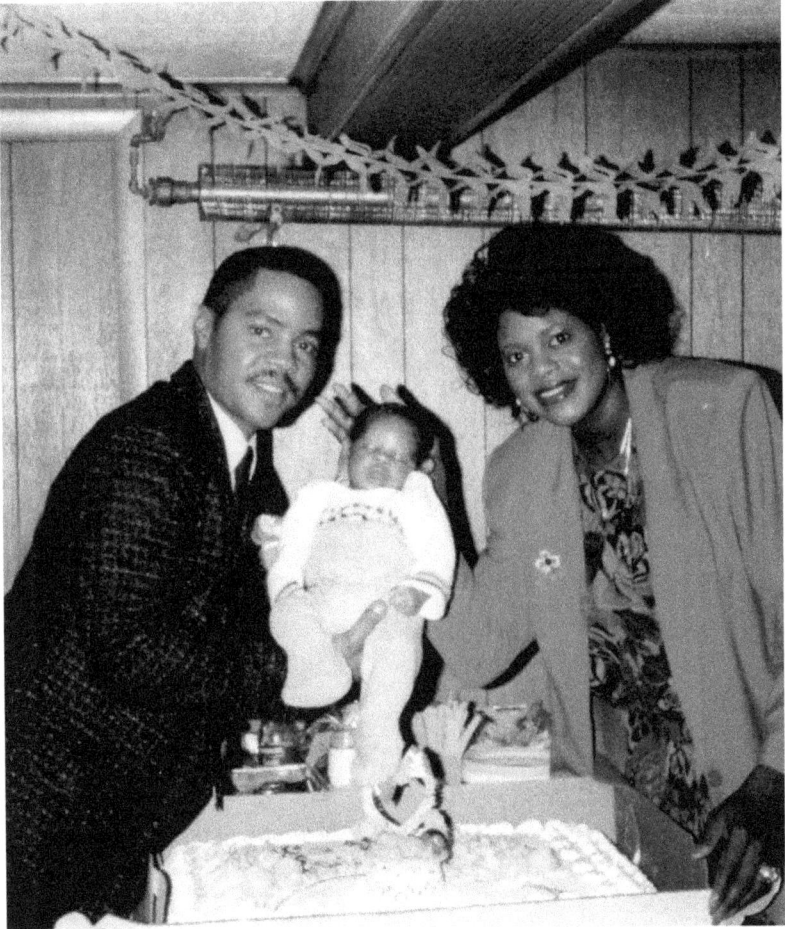

Christening Day and Baby Shower - March 16, 1991
Melvin, Christopher, and I at my parent's house.

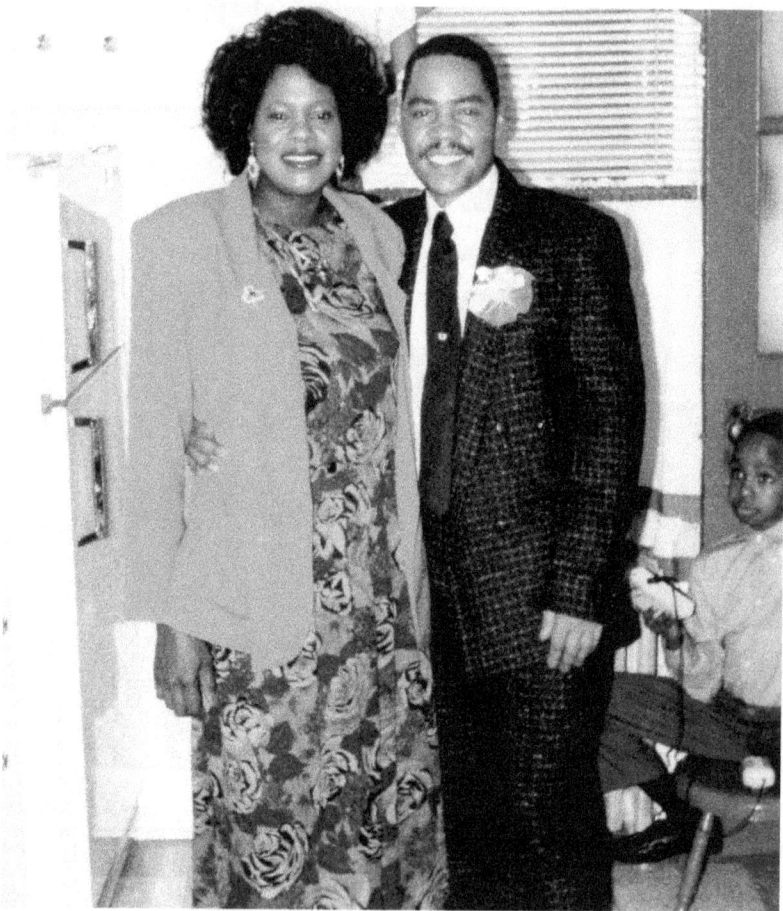

Melvin and I in the kitchen, and my nephew, Jason in the background - March 16, 1991.

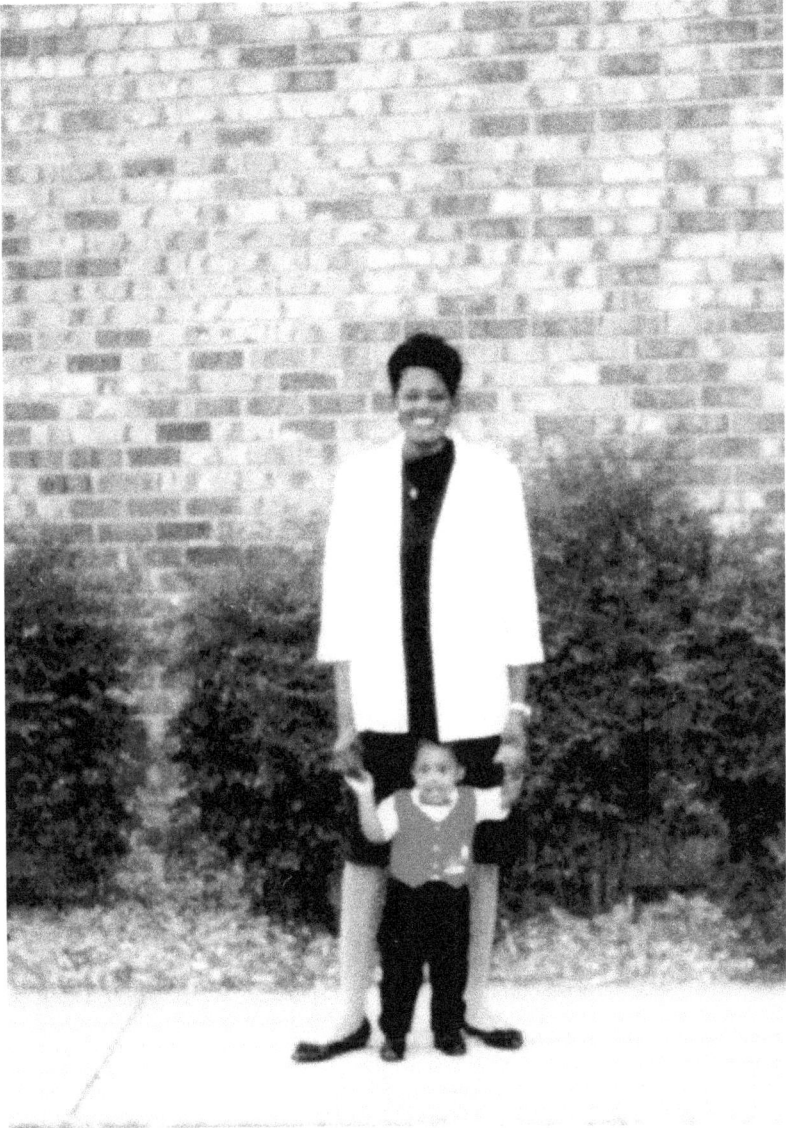

Easter weekend in Atlanta - 1992. My son and I in front of the Days Inn.

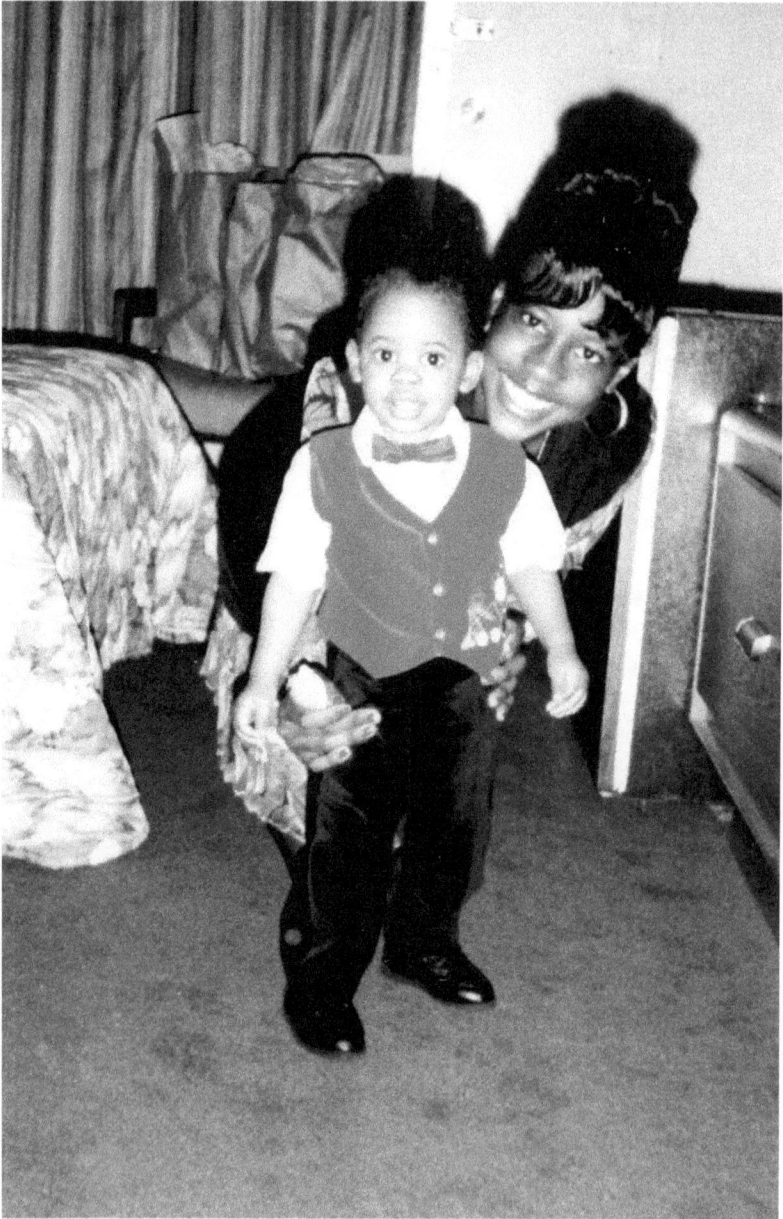

My daughter, Christine and my son, Christopher at the Days Inn.

PART II

LIVING
IN
ATLANTA

CHAPTER 6

MY ARRIVAL

I could not believe that, all on June 27, 1992, I made forty years old, was five months pregnant, and had just moved to Atlanta, Georgia. After we arrived in Atlanta, we took a taxi to our new home. As we were pulling up to the front of the driveway, we saw a very long truck slowly coming up the street. To our surprise, the moving truck was pulling up at the exact same time as us. The drivers told us that they got lost along the way. We told them that it was perfect timing because we had missed our flight. I told them that if we would have come the day that we were scheduled to arrive there would not have been a bed for me to sleep in and no cars for us to get around in. So, everything worked out for the best, and I was able to enjoy a very happy birthday!

Something Is Just Not Right!

As we were opening the door to the new house, Melvin was carefully looking around and checking things out. I was showing the movers where everything should go. After we were in the house, Melvin told me that the house was haunted. I looked at him like he was crazy. I completely ignored what he had said to me. I thought to myself, *Is he just saying that because he wants us to go back home to New York City?* But, he insisted that he was not kidding.

"The house is haunted. I know you don't believe me because we just got here, but I'm telling you, this house is really haunted!" He said. He told me that when he went downstairs to the basement, he opened the basement door and saw a man running to the back of the room. But, when he went to look, there was no sign of the man anywhere. He said that all of a sudden the windows started opening up all by themselves and a voice shouted to him saying, "Get Out!"

Once we got settled, we started to see that Melvin's personality was changing all of a sudden and we did not know why. My daughter and I said that he was such a nice person when we lived in New York, but now that we were living in Georgia, we did not know what was bringing all of this on. After a short time had passed, Melvin told me that he needed to get back to New York. I said, "Get back to New York?" I couldn't believe it! I was so mad at him that I told him to just go. He began getting himself together, packing his things, and he drove all the way back to New York.

After he was back in New York, he persistently called, telling me that he wanted to come back to Georgia. So, after talking things over and clearing the air with him, he drove himself all the way back to Georgia. Soon after he got back, I began having dreams about him that something was not right. I felt that there was something bothering him really bad inside. He also looked so disgusted and puzzled with himself and I was wondering what could be going on. I knew that it was definitely not me. I could not figure out what the problem was.

Finally, Melvin could not take it any longer and told me what had happened. I could not believe what I was hearing. He told me that his ex-wife was pregnant.

"What! When did all of this happen?" I questioned.

"Remember the time that we had an argument back in New York and I left?"

"Yeah." I answered.

"I was so angry that I just decided to stay at my ex-wife's house. Then, after you and I talked things over, I came back." He explained. I was so angry! I started adding up the time in my head and that meant that his ex-wife and I were both one month apart from each other. She was due in September and I was due in October.

"Oh, what a big mess you've created for yourself!" I said. That hurt me too much. I told him that I did not want to deal with it, so the best thing for him to do, at that point, was to take all of his stuff and go back to New York.

"The worst thing about it is, if I would have known sooner, I would have never moved to Atlanta. I sacrificed everything to come and live in this new state." I told him.

He continued to tell me that his ex-wife did not tell him anything about the pregnancy until after we moved to Atlanta because she did not want to mess up his plans. He told me that as if it was supposed to make me feel better. I was definitely not mad at her one bit because I had no idea what he was telling her. None of that even mattered to me. It was the fact that we were both pregnant. I found myself put in a really bad situation and I had to think things through really fast! I already knew that when my baby was born, I would have a very tough road ahead of me. But, I knew deep in my heart that I would be okay.

There were some people that I had already met in Georgia, both men and women that had extended themselves out to me because I was pregnant. They gave me their telephone numbers and said that they would be more than willing to take me to the hospital, day or night when I was in labor. I appreciated that very much. Christine was hoping that I would have the baby on the weekend. That way, she would not have to miss time away from school.

I Was in Labor

It was around 1:40 AM and I was in labor. I felt bad needing to do this, but I had to call my beautician to ask if she could take me to the hospital. After I called her, I could not believe how fast she rushed over to my house. She took me straight downtown to Grady Memorial Hospital. When we arrived, she told the doctors that she would not be staying because she already knew that my baby was going to be born in just a few short hours. The doctor immediately started checking me and said, "Yes, your baby is definitely ready." I thanked her so much for bringing me to the hospital. She told me not to worry, that I would be okay, and then she left.

My Baby Was Born

The doctor who was going to deliver my baby let me know that she needed to get something and would be right back. At that time, there were nurses in the room assisting me. When my doctor came back, to her surprise, she saw my baby's head starting to come out. With a few good pushes, my baby was born. That was my easiest delivery.

My little girl was born on October 24, 1992, at 4:06 AM. She weighed 6 lbs. 11oz., and was 19 inches long. My little girl and I have the same blood type. Her first name is Christel, which is still the first name that carries from Dr. Christine Lawrence in New York—the doctor I was seeing for my lupus at the Arthritis Clinic in New York, while I was pregnant, was Dr. Betty Diamond. I gave my baby girl my doctor's last name by using it for her middle name. Therefore, my baby girl's full name is Christel Diamond Bethune. What a pretty name she has! I have been fortunate enough to have excellent doctors to help me throughout my life. And, despite having lupus, I was extremely blessed to have had three beautiful children. I was so happy!

After my baby was born and I was resting in my hospital room, I made it known to the nurses that I did not have any family members here in Georgia and that I would be leaving the hospital alone with my baby. They told me not to worry about anything while I was there and that they would take good care of me. And they did just that. I felt so great and did not feel lonely one bit. All I have to say is that I had a beautiful delivery and an excellent stay at Grady Memorial Hospital.

I was also happy that my daughter was able to get her wish. Christine's little baby sister was born on the weekend just like she wanted.

Soon after the birth of little Christel, Melvin drove back to Atlanta and made sure that his daughter's birth certificate records were completely updated with his name and information on it. He spent quality time with his children. On Saturday January 9, 1993, my children's dad left to go back to New York.

Christel's Ears Were Being Pierced

On March 7, 1993, when my little girl Christel was four months old, I decided that I would like to have her ears pierced. I took her to the store near where I lived. The lady was able to pierce her ears without any problem. It was done so fast! After that, I always kept her cute, little tiny, gold loop earrings in her ears.

Seeking Employment

Since Christel was born, six months ago, my health had been good. I started seeking employment opportunities. On April 5, 1993, I started a medical transcriptionist position near the airport. I was working in a very fast paced environment, which consisted of completing medical reports that had been dictated on tapes from doctors. I had never done that type of work before, so I knew that it was going to be very challenging for me. Since all of the work was being timed, you also had to understand the medical terminology, which definitely could slow you down a bit if you didn't. So, the faster I completed the reports for the doctors, the more money I made. I knew that this type of job was too stressful and not for me at all, so I immediately moved on from it.

My youngest children's dad, Melvin, was constantly calling us from New York and wanted so much to be back in Georgia. I was thinking, *Here we go again!* When the month of May came, their dad was so happy to be back. I felt much better because he was making an effort to be in their lives.

I met a young lady when I was at the paint store one day; her name was Beth Carter. I was looking for paint and wallpaper that I could install myself. I was able to find what I needed and could not wait to put it up. Beth saw how knowledgeable I was. She said that she was buying a very large quantity of wallpaper that she was going to install herself in beautiful mansions where her clients lived. She let me know that she could use a little help installing wallpaper. I did not know where my life was headed at that moment, but I decided to work with her.

After being on the jobsite with her a few times, and seeing the type of work that she was doing in those mansions, it was definitely a bit too much for me. When Beth told me that some of the jobs consisted of having to use scaffolds, I knew it was definitely not for me.

Immediately after that, Melvin was able to get a job working for a roofing company. He was not familiar at all with the Atlanta area, but took a job with a very, very long commute that really wiped him out.

The last two weeks in May was very busy for me. I was running around with my daughter, Christine. She was heavily involved in all of the extracurricular activities in her school—which consisted of a great deal of evening rehearsals and preparing for an upcoming performance being held in June.

After a few weeks went by, everything seemed to be going fine. However, Melvin still looked so confused. He started telling me, once again, that he could no longer be in Georgia with us. He said that the house was telling him to get out.

"Get out?" I questioned.

"Yes! The house said, 'Get out. Get the hell out!'" He claimed. He said that the house told him that if he does not get out, he will be sorry. "Boo, Boo"—the name he used to call me—"I have to leave. I know you don't believe me Boo, Boo, but one day you will see that I was telling you the truth."

I really did not understand any of it. I did not know what in the world was going on with him. None of it made any sense to me anymore. I thought, *Why in the world would he keep driving back and forth, from New York to Georgia, when he has no intentions of staying?* So, on Sunday June 6, 1993, Melvin left once again to go right back to New York.

Now that he had arrived back in New York, he tried

to explain his reasoning. At that point, I didn't even care. I did not want to talk or even listen to what he had to say. I was just too mad at him. He knew that I had no intentions of coming back to New York City to live because I had invested too much in Georgia. In the meantime, it was definitely time for me to move on with my life and his two young children, without him.

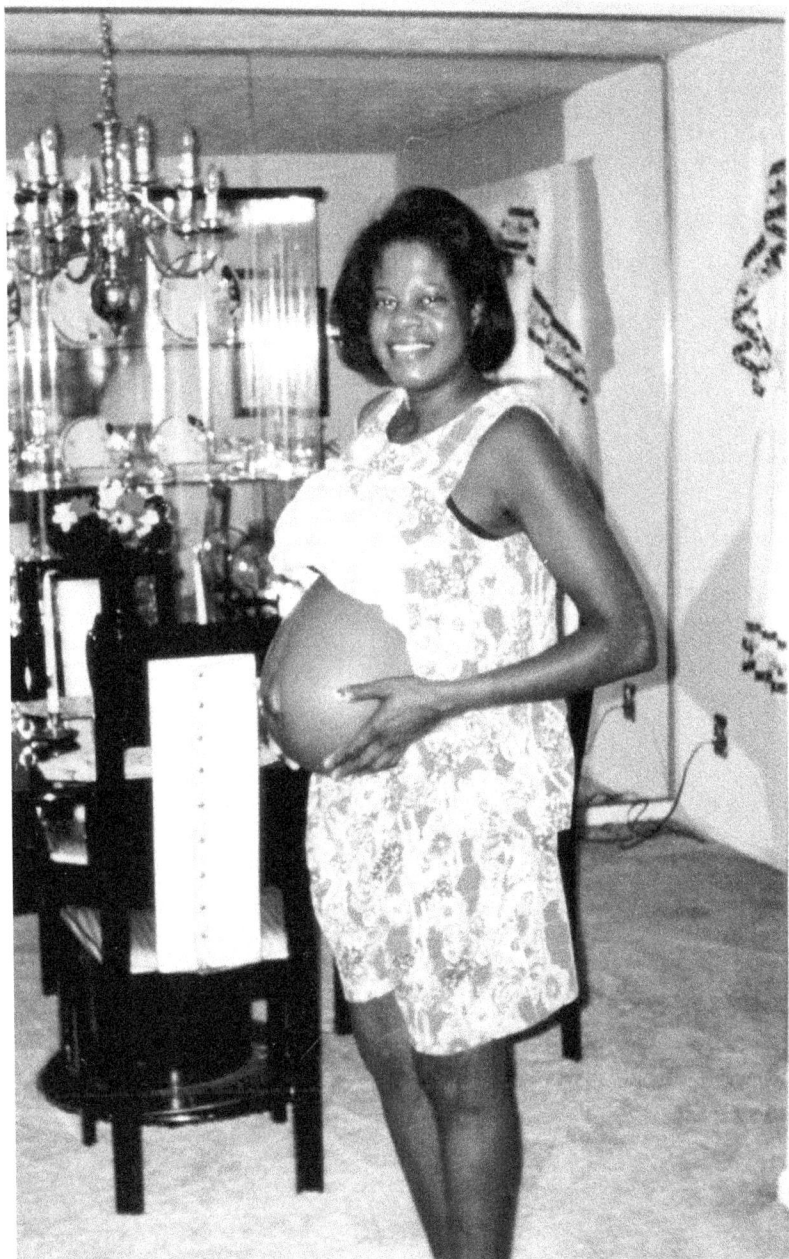

At home. I was pregnant with my baby girl.

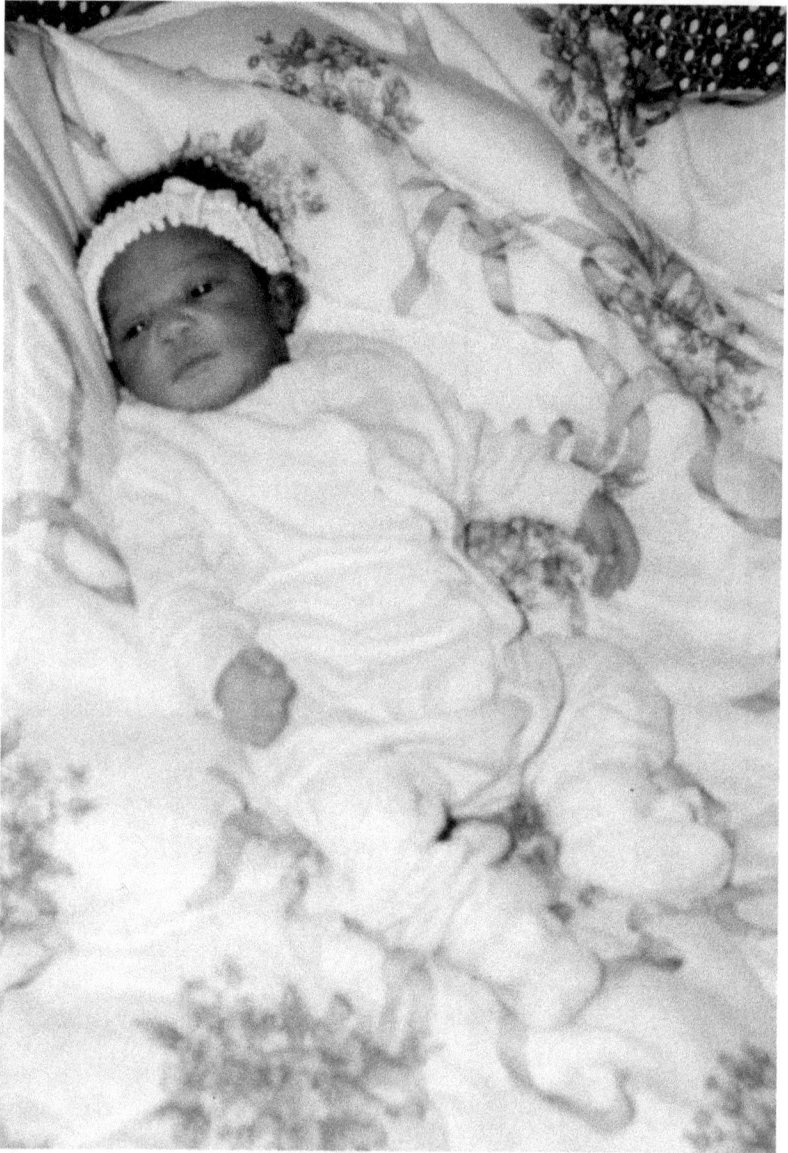

My daughter, Christel Diamond Bethune at home. She was three days old.

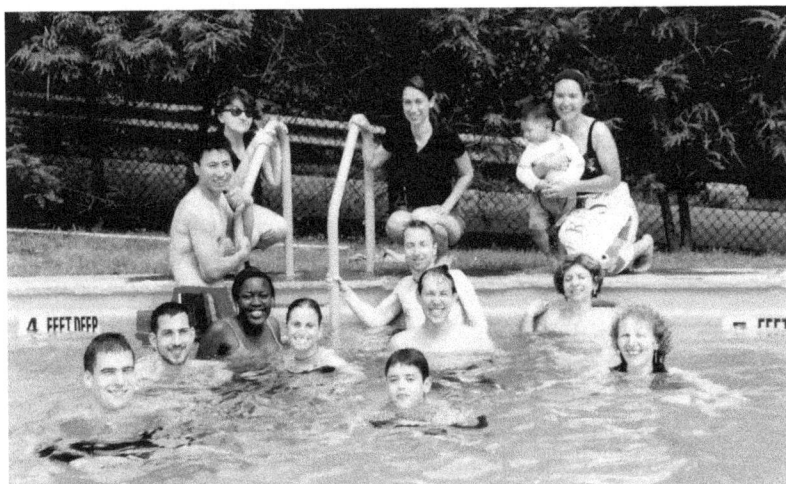

Front far right: Dr. Betty Diamond and her lab were in a park for a lab party.

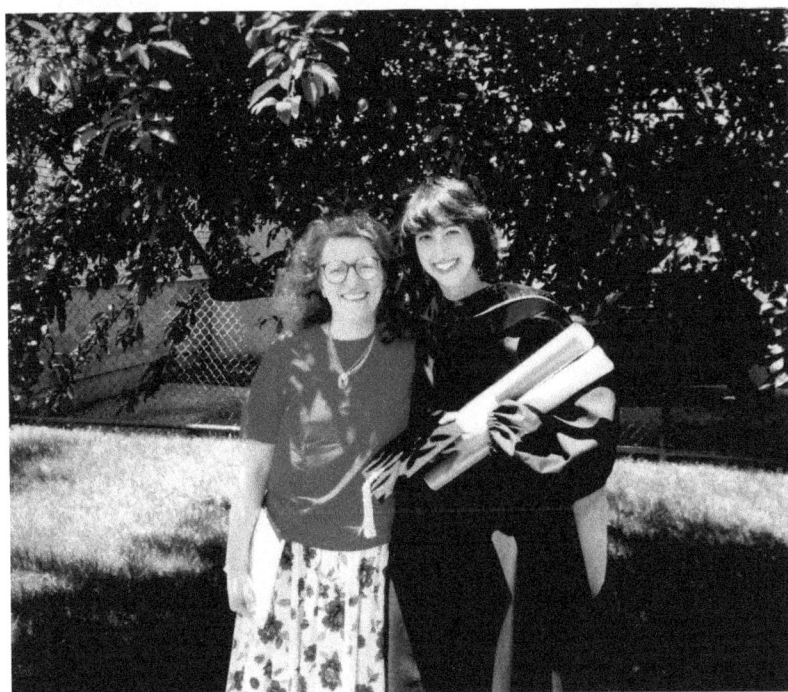

Dr. Betty Diamond and a student receiving her PhD. Student now works at Harvard studying kidney disease.

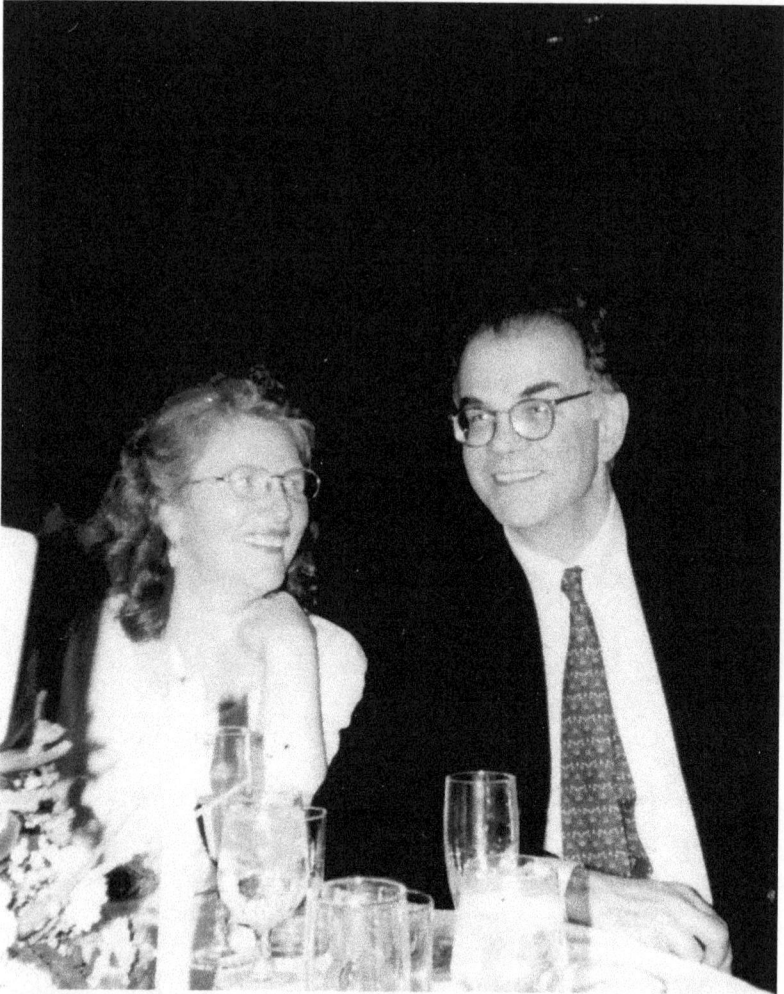

Dr. Betty Diamond and her husband at an SLE Foundation Gala to raise money for lupus research.

CHAPTER 7

FACING CHALLENGES

I was a mother of three, living on my own, in another state, and trying to make it all happen. I knew that it was not going to be easy for me. It was one of the hardest challenges in my life that I had to face. I knew in my heart that I am a very strong person, and that I would keep on striving to get through all of this. Looking at my three beautiful children was what kept me going.

Christel's Baptism

It was a beautiful Sunday morning on July 18, 1993, and my little girl, Christel Diamond Bethune, was getting baptized. Her baptism was being held at New Life A.M.E. Zion Church in College Park, Georgia. My family was in attendance from New York City. I was so grateful for their support to be with us and will always cherish the memories.

At the Unemployment Office

Come August of 1993, I knew that I had to do something different because time was running out. I tried to think fast and hard about what to do for income. I decided to go to the unemployment office. I was determined to find something that day. While I was there, the office was making an announcement. They had openings for jobs! They informed us about a security company that was looking for people who could start working immediately. They said that whoever was interested in a position should please head on up to the front desk. I was too happy after hearing the announcement and came straight up. After being interviewed, I was hired.

I immediately called my mom and dad. "You will be working the grave yard shift?" My father asked concerned. I told him that I would only stay for a short period of time until I found something else. After working nights for about two weeks, I realized that shift just did not work for me. I did not like the fact that my teenage daughter was home alone. So, I stopped working with that company. When it comes to my three children, I do whatever it takes to make sure that they are always okay, and if it doesn't look like it is going to work out like it should, at least I can say that I tried.

Christine and Christopher's Godmother Was Visiting – 8/17/93

Since I was not working at the time, Christine and Christopher's godmother, Aunt Abie, knew what I was going through. She had some vacation time from her job, so she decided she would come to Atlanta and spend some time with us. She arrived in Atlanta on August 17, 1993 at 9:50 PM. We were very happy to see her.

When I first took Abie down to the basement, she really loved the size of it. She immediately asked me, "Valerie what is that smell?"

"What smell?" I replied.

She said, "I smell moth balls." I told her that I put a few moth balls in the back closet during the summer months because I was getting moths. She started looking at me funny. She told me that those moth balls were really strong. She said that it felt like it was stifling her and making it hard for her to breathe. She said, "I'm getting out of this basement." She left the basement as fast as she could. Once she got out, she said, "I can breathe now." I was surprised that it got to her like that.

During her stay, I took her downtown where she was able to tour the birth home of Dr. Martin Luther King, Jr. She enjoyed going to the Underground. We ate out a lot and just enjoyed being with one another. Abie left Atlanta on Monday, August 23, 1993 at 1:10 PM and arrived in New York at 4:49 PM. She said that she had a great time and loved being in Atlanta.

Christopher and Christel in Day Care

One day, when I was in the food store, I was fortunate enough to meet a lady who owned her own day care center. I shared my situation with her. She encouraged me to start my own day care, but I had not intended on doing that. I told her that I was seeking employment and needed to put my two young children in day care while I go on job interviews. I could not believe it, but she told me that she would take care of my two children free of charge.

My two children were in day care as 'drop-ins' only until I found employment. I was so grateful for that. They stayed at that day care for about three visits. On that last visit, I dropped them off in the morning and my son started having a temper tantrum. I felt so bad. He just cried and cried.

When I arrived to pick up my son and daughter, my son was so happy to see me. He wanted to get out of that day care fast. While we were walking to my car, I noticed that my son was looking at me and shivering. As I picked him up and put him in his car seat, I could not believe how soaking wet his clothes were—even with his jacket on! I was so angry that I wanted to turn around, go back inside, and show them just how soaking wet he was. But, due to the fact that I was not a paying client, I dare not go back. It was one of the lady's workers who was supposed to be taking care of him. She definitely was not being responsible enough while my son was in her care. I immediately opened my trunk, found some plastic bags, and put them in his car seat. My son started crying because he was so wet and shaking his head as I drove away. He was letting me know that he did not want to go back there again.

When we arrived home, I immediately took them out of their car seats, went upstairs, and took their wet clothes off. After giving them their nice warm baths, they felt so happy. I gave them a great big hug and a kiss on their little cheeks. I told my son, "Christopher, you will not be going back there again."

Changing My Life's Plan

After my son's traumatic episode in day care, I had to quickly change my life's plan. So, during the latter part of September 1993, I was seriously thinking about starting my own in-home child care. I was a little scared because it was definitely out of my comfort zone. My sister, Claudette's, best friend, Beverly, told me that I would make a wonderful child care provider. I had been in the legal field for so many years. That meant facing the fact that the type of jobs I did while living in New York City with only one child, I could no longer do while living in Georgia as a single parent and raising three children.

It was very expensive putting my two youngest children in day care, and I was trying to figure things out for myself and my children. Therefore, I became a state certified child care provider. I was providing care on a part-time basis at that time. I needed to be as flexible as possible for my three children. My oldest daughter was always extremely involved in so many extracurricular activities at her school. She also had to rehearse for a big drama performance during late October 1993. She was really happy to be a part of the show, but that meant driving her back and forth each day.

Changing the Way I Receive Child Support

During the time of December 1993, I decided that, rather than having Melvin send his child support monies directly to me, I preferred that he send it straight to the court. That way, anything that he sent would be fully documented. At that time, monies had not been consistent because he was a construction worker and was not able to work in inclement weather.

Inspiration from Everyone

Since my children's dad had left, I was receiving inspirational letters from everyone that I had been in contact with. I received a beautiful letter from my youngest sister's best friend that was dated December 10, 1993. In her letter, she stated that she believed in God and knew that he puts no more on us than we can bear. The letter of encouragement was very nice.

Strange Things Were Happening

The year of 1994, made two years that we had been living in Georgia. Strange things were happening in my home around the same time that my youngest sister, Claudette and her son, Jason, were visiting us.

One morning, when I was going into the kitchen to use the microwave, I opened the microwave door, and I could not believe what I saw…there were millions of ants on the inside of the microwave, just crawling around. I yelled out to everyone to come and look at all of these ants in the microwave! My microwave was very clean before we all went to bed last night, so I could not understand where all of the ants came from. And, why were they just crawling on the inside of the microwave and nowhere else? That seemed so crazy to me.

There was another strange incident that happened during the time Claudette and I went to the store to buy a few things. While at the store, I saw some beautiful fake red roses that I liked, so I purchased them. When we returned home, I put the fake flowers in my beautiful black vase and placed it on the dining room table.

After we started putting things away, Claudette and I decided to call our father at home in New York City because we knew he was not feeling well. When we called, our dad picked up the telephone and spoke with both of us. He told us that our mom was at the senior citizen center at that time. As the conversation continued, he suddenly asked us, "Who is eating peppermint?"

"Peppermint!" We said, "Dad, no one is eating any peppermint!"

"I am telling you, I smell peppermint!" My dad said that the smell of peppermint was coming through his telephone very strong. Claudette and I were both looking at each other in amazement, as we could hear the frustration in our dad's voice. We could not believe what he was saying to us. We did not smell anything. We decided that our dad was just not feeling well, and we cut the conversation short until our mom came home. We told our dad to get some rest and that we would call him back later that night. He said that was okay.

Claudette and I hung up the telephone and stayed in the kitchen. After that, we started smelling peppermint. It was getting stronger and stronger. The kitchen and the dining room were in two separate rooms, but right next to each other. We followed the smell that was leading us into the dining room. Not only were the fake flowers that I bought smelling up the whole dining room like peppermint, but the red roses were dripping all over the table like blood. We said, "Oh my goodness! Dad was right!" My sister and I were shocked!

"How in the world did Dad smell peppermint all the way from New York City?" I said to my sister. We just could not believe it.

"When you were buying those flowers, Valerie, something about them just didn't look right to me. I knew how much you liked them, so I just didn't say anything." My sister told me.

"They didn't look strange to me at all. I liked them because they were different. Just big beautiful red roses with little clear plastic rain drops on them. That's what I liked about them."

My sister and I had to get those flowers back to the store before it closed for the night. As I picked up that black vase with those big red roses in it, the roses dripped all over my light-colored carpet. We headed down the stairs to the garage where my car was parked. I could not do anything about the stains at that exact moment because it was getting late and we had to get to the store before it closed.

When we arrived at the store, I spoke with customer service and they could see from the receipt that those roses were just purchased. I told them everything that had happened. The employees could not believe that the red roses smelled like peppermint and dripped like blood.

I was able to get my money back. The store assured me that they would gladly put a claim in for me for the damages that were done to my carpet floor. They were all very nice about everything. I was told to come back the next morning so that they could take care of everything. We were glad to get rid of those flowers. What a relief that was.

When we returned back home, I immediately checked to see which floors had stains on them. As I looked around, I said, "Oh, No! This cannot be." I told my sister to come and look because all of the stains had disappeared. Everything on that carpet was gone. I wanted to know where all of the stains went. There were no signs of peppermint smell in the house at all. It was like nothing ever happened.

We called our mom and dad back and told them what had happened. We told our dad that he was right and that it was the fake flowers I had purchased. He said, "See, I told you I was right. Y'all thought I was crazy."

I said, "Wow, all of this is so weird to me!" I told my sister that I would not be going back to the store that following day to submit the claim. I told her that I would just call back and tell them that the stains came out and just leave it like that.

After that drastic episode, everything was back to normal and Claudette and Jason's visit was enjoyable.

My Stepbrother's Passing – 11/11/94

My oldest stepbrother, Alonzo Colley, became suddenly ill during September 1987. He became stricken by a mysterious paralyzing illness that took him to so many hospitals and nursing homes. The sad part of it all was that no one was able to find out what caused his illness or find a cure. He later passed away on November 11, 1994.

Child Support Payments Were Not Up to Date

On November 15, 1994, I contacted child support collections informing them that I had spoken with my two youngest children's father in March and that the last child support payment I received from him was on March 29, 1994. Too many months had now gone by. Therefore, I was sent an application regarding the matter.

Claudette and Jason Moved to Atlanta

During late December 1994, just before New Year's, my youngest sister, Claudette and her son, Jason moved to Atlanta and stayed with us until they got settled.

Registering Christopher into the Head Start Program

My little boy, Christopher, was growing up so nicely. When it was January 9, 1995, I registered him into the J.F. Beavers' Clark Atlanta University's Head Start

Program. Christopher had always been a focused young boy who was ready and willing to learn new and exciting things. That Head Start Program was going to be a great new start for him. He will be able to interact with children his own age, thus preparing him for kindergarten.

That first day of school, for Christopher, was a little sad. He was so used to being at home with me. When we were driving in the car and we pulled up in front of the school, his face completely changed. After he saw all of the little boys and girls, his eyes just lit up as he started smiling. I did not have to worry. I knew that he was going to have a very nice first day at school.

When I returned to pick Christopher up, the teachers told me that he was such a very nice, well-behaved little boy and that it was a pleasure having him in their class. He was so happy that he started showing me all of the things he had done that day. He continued to look forward to his days at school.

Lupus Flare-up - 1/27/95

I had been doing really well for myself, and I have not had a lupus flare-up for quite some time. But, on January 27, 1995, I had a doctor's appointment at the W.T. Brooks Clinic and the doctor had to start me on three 5 mg Prednisone pills daily.

On Sunday, February 5, 1995 Claudette and I went out. We were seated near an entrance doorway that was very drafty. That following day, I started getting sick. I experienced very bad pains in the back of my neck, as well as some cramps in my legs.

Things continued to get worse. I woke up with very severe pain throughout my body. My knees were swollen with inflammation. My hands were tight and so badly swollen that it was hard for me to write. To say the least, my entire body ached. I noticed that my hair was also falling out.

Being Referred to Grady Memorial Hospital's Rheumatology Clinic

When I went to the W.T. Brooks Clinic on that Wednesday morning, February 8, 1995, my doctor kept me on that same dose of Prednisone. My urine had traces of blood in it, which did not end up being serious. My doctor took blood tests, gave me a breast exam, and a pap test, which all came back normal. After looking through my records, the doctor felt that the clinic had done the best that they could do during the time I had been receiving treatment there. Since further testing needed to be done for my lupus, the clinic referred me to Grady Memorial Hospital. From there, I would continue to receive the necessary treatment. It would give me an opportunity to see how other lupus patients have also been dealing with this dreadful disease.

Rheumatology Clinic Appointments

During the time of March 1995, I was being seen at Grady Memorial Hospital's Rheumatology Clinic. For that second week in March, I had to alternate taking three 5 mg Prednisone pills on one day, and then the next day taking two 5 mg Prednisone pills. I had to repeat that method until my next appointment in April.

On April 24, 1995, I had a 9:00 AM doctor's appointment at Grady Memorial Hospital. I was seen at their Rheumatology Clinic. During that visit, the doctor informed me that things were progressing a little better for me.

Child Support Proceedings Had Begun

When it was April 27, 1995, child support proceedings had begun for my two youngest children.

Claudette's Life Was About to Change

One day, my youngest sister, Claudette and I decided that we would go apartment hunting. As we were driving around, Claudette saw a very nice apartment complex that she really liked. When we went in and to her surprise the apartment that she was interested in was available. After the leasing office went over everything with her, she was able to get the apartment.

During that same week, Claudette also had a job interview. The company was very interested in her and she was offered a receptionist position. She could not believe how everything happened so quickly—all in the same week! I was very happy for my sister's brand new start in Atlanta, and that her new life was about to change in a positive way.

Dermatology Clinic

On May 8, 1995, I had a 9:00 AM appointment at the Dermatology Clinic at Grady Memorial Hospital. I was breaking out with a rash on my cheeks.

The Teacher Who Made a Difference in My Daughter, Christine's Life

When my daughter, Christine, was attending Tri-Cities High School for the Visual and Performing Arts, it gave her a very active social life and so much more to look forward to. Her drama teacher, Mr. Hendricks, was the one who made the biggest impact in my daughter's life. He was a very inspirational teacher, as well as a mentor to her. I am so proud of what she accomplished there.

When it was May 1995, the end of the school year was approaching. Christine wanted so much to attend her high school prom. It was held on May 20, 1995. Christine was extremely excited. Before rushing out, my sister helped drape my daughter's long, silver scarf around the top of her dress.

Lupus Flare-up – 5/25/95

On the morning of May 25, 1995, I was seen at 8:15 AM at the Rheumatology Clinic at Grady. At that time, my doctor said that he would increase my Prednisone just a little. He instructed me ahead of time that when Saturday came, June 3, 1995, I would need to increase my Prednisone to three and a half 5 mg pills daily. That meant that my face was going to be round and puffy-looking for my daughter's graduation day. During the months following, I was given careful instructions on how my Prednisone medication should be slowly decreased until I was seen again in September.

Christine's Graduation – Seventeen Years Old

It was time for my seventeen-year-old daughter, Christine to graduate. My mother came down from New York City to be with us, as well as my ex-husband's family from Mobile, Alabama. Christine's graduation exercises were held at Tri-Cities High School Stadium on Saturday, June 10, 1995, at 7:00 PM. The graduation ceremony turned out very nice. Christine received many awards for all of her accomplishments. After the ceremony was over, we were all invited back to a very nice reception at Christine's friend's house where we stayed for the rest of the evening.

Child Support Review

On August 15, 1995, I received a letter from child support services. They advised me of my right to request that they review my most recent child support order to determine whether it should be changed to require health insurance for my daughter. If I wished to request a review of the child support order, it must be made in writing.

I promptly responded back to their request, in writing, on September 1, 1995. Christine had not been receiving any health insurance from her father for the past thirteen years.

My Doctors Appointments - New Medication

During the month of September 1995, when I was seen at Grady Memorial Hospital, the doctor decided to put me on a new medication called Hydroxychloroquine at 200 mgs. My Prednisone had already been decreased, and I was taking only one pill each day. I saw the doctor again in October.

Well, after I had used the new medication, I definitely did not like the way it made me feel. It made my eyes feel so heavy; all I wanted to do was just close them and go right to sleep—which I often did. That was not a good feeling at all and it took all of my energy away. I was never the type of person who just wanted to sleep all day. So, on my next appointment—which was October 25, 1995—I immediately told the doctor about Hydroxychloroquine and how it made me feel and was told to discontinue using it. At the time of my visit, I was only taking one 5 mg Prednisone pill daily—which was really good—one 25 mg Hydrochlorothiazide water pill daily, a Potassium pill K-DUR 20 MEQ - 1500 mgs. I had to take that pill once daily with plenty of water. I also took a 325 mg pill of Ferrous Sulfate.

When the month of November came, my Prednisone had to be slightly changed. I was so used to taking 5 mg pills, but now I had to take 1 mg Prednisone pills.

Therefore, my 1 mg Prednisone pills were taken this way: I had to take eight 1 mg pills daily for two weeks, then seven 1 mg pills daily for two weeks, then six 1 mg pills daily for two weeks, and finally I had to stay on a total of five 1 mg pills daily until I was seen at my next doctor's appointment.

At the beginning of the New Year, 1996, I was forty-three years old. That was the year that I was seriously thinking about moving out of the house where my children and I had been living.

I did see my doctor on January 23, 1996. I was advised to take one Potassium pill K-DUR 20 MEQ - 1500 mgs daily. Other than that, everything else was fine.

My Father's Passing

My father had been sick for quite some time. On Thursday, February 8, 1996, he passed away. My father was born on December 25, 1921 (Christmas Day) in White Springs, Florida. On February 14, 1996 (Valentine's Day) my father was buried.

My father was a United States Army veteran, serving in the Asiatic Pacific Theater in World War II. He was a recipient of two Bronze Service Stars, Good Conduct Medal and Victory Medal. After thirty years of occupational service with the City of New York, my father retired. He was a jack-of-all-trades. He enjoyed traveling and always took time out of his busy schedule to help others.

My father was a wonderful person to all of us. We miss him dearly. We will always remember those beautiful memories and the times we shared with him.

A Letter from the Court

I was so happy that, after sometime had passed, I received a letter from the court dated February 23, 1996. They were writing to see if changes should be made to require health insurance for my daughter, Christine Horn. I submitted my yearly income tax to the court on March 5, 1996 and was waiting to hear back from them.

Bed Wetting

When my son, Christopher was four years old, he still did not like sleeping in his own bed at night; he was constantly wetting the bed. I had to always make sure that I did not give him any fluids prior to his bedtime. He would tell me that he was not going to wet his bed, but he continued to do it. I always kept a night light on in the hall so that he would not be scared to use the bathroom.

Strange Things Continued to Happen

My sister and her son had already moved into their own apartment, but strange things continued to happen at my house. One Sunday morning, around 10:30 AM, my children and I were ready to leave the house for the 11:00 AM church service. As we were headed downstairs to the basement area that leads to the garage, the garage door would not open. It felt as if someone was holding onto the door so tight that I could not even open it. I was pulling and banging on the door and nothing was happening. I was so angry that we were missing church service.

So, the first thing that came to my mind was to immediately call the last owners who lived there. I wanted to see if they had ever experienced anything like that. The wife was the one who answered the telephone. I told her exactly what I was going through. She honestly told me that sometimes she would hear people playing basketball in the garage. She said that she would be so scared because she knew that she was the only one at home. She said that when she went to look in the garage, there was nobody there. She admitted that this was the reason why they decided to have an alarm system put in. She also said that, since her husband had to travel out of town a lot, the alarm system made her feel safe and so much better living there.

After that, she told me that was not the only reason for their leaving. She told me that when she would go in the backyard, there would always be so many bats flying around and that really scared her. So, she felt that she could not stay there anymore. Her husband told me that his wife would always say things to him about what she was going through, but he said that he never experienced anything while he was living there. He said that he had really good luck when he lived there.

After hearing all of that, I told Christopher and Christel that we had to forget about going to church that Sunday because it was getting too late. I explained to them that, since the garage door was not opening up for us, we would just take off our church clothes and relax in the family room. All of a sudden, around 1:00 PM, I heard the heating system come on with a full blast of air. I jumped off the couch to see what was happening. The doors leading down to the basement burst open all by themselves. I was so scared. I never witnessed anything like that in my life. I thought to myself, *This house does not want me to go to church, so it let the doors open when it knew that my church service was about over.* I did not feel good about what was going on in that house.

There was another time when I was watching television in the family room and, seated near the entranceway that leads right out into the hall, I had the strangest feeling that someone was watching me from behind. As I quickly turned around to check, there was a nice looking white man with his legs crossed, leaning by the gate in the hall that leads downstairs to the front entrance door. I was too scared to say anything to the man because I could not believe what I was seeing and my front entrance door was closed. I was thinking to myself, *Where did this man come from?* He was looking directly at me without blinking—just staring at me. I turned my head away from him and then quickly turned back around to see if he was still there. He had disappeared!

A Description of the Man

He was a nice looking white man with a clean-shaven face. He was slim, but not too tall. He was wearing a white short-sleeved T-shirt that was tucked inside of his gray dress pants. He wore a black belt around his waist and black dress shoes. His hair was low cut, and he seemed to have been in his 30's to mid-40's.

After seeing what I saw, that was definitely the last straw for me. I could not stand it any longer. Things were getting creepier and creepier by the day, and I wanted my children out of there!

Thank goodness my children were napping and my oldest daughter was always busy with extracurricular activities, so she never experienced anything while living in that house. Lucky for her! It was time for me to start looking for a new place to live.

Time to Look for a Broker

I knew it was time for me to look for a broker. So one Friday evening, when I was looking through the newspaper, I felt that whichever broker's ad hits me right in the face and sounded good to me would be the one who I would definitely use to sell my house. I was able to find a very large and striking ad and immediately called Daphne. We decided to meet first thing that following Monday morning.

After Daphne arrived, we sat down at the kitchen table and went over all the particulars. A few days later, my home had been listed, and I looked forward to getting it sold.

My Open House

The day before my Open House, it had been raining all day long until midnight. I went downstairs to the basement and there was so much water coming into the basement. It was so bad that Christine and I had to put our boots on and start shoveling out the water. At that moment I did not know what else to do! I needed to call Daphne, but it was too late. So, I told my daughter, Christine, that I would wait and cancel the Open House in the morning.

Wow! I could not believe what I saw. The morning of my Open House, I went downstairs to the basement to see how much water was still there. I was so shocked! All of the water that was in the basement was totally gone. There were no signs of water anywhere. That was so crazy! I could not wait for Daphne to arrive so I could tell her everything that had happened. My house was definitely going to sell. The backyard was very big and had a very large swimming pool.

When it was time for the Open House, there were a number of brokers and their clients touring my home. We received positive feedback from everyone. On one of the house showings, there was a very nice interracial couple that came with their broker to see the house. I did not know what was happening at that time, but my doors, blinds, and windows were closed and the blinds suddenly started clattering back and forth. The couple's broker was startled by that. She looked at the windows and quietly whispered to her clients, "Let's get out of here, this house is haunted." I thought to myself, *She felt the house was haunted?* What was so amazing to me was that it only happened to that one broker. As quickly as all of that happened, we found a buyer for my house immediately! The only problem was, I had two weeks to find another place to live.

So, Daphne and I went to look at some houses. I did not see anything that I was interested in and I was discouraged. I told Daphne that if I did not find a house in that short amount of time, I was willing to settle for an apartment. Daphne told me that she did not want me to settle for an apartment because my money would dwindle away really fast. She told me to do whatever I had to do to make sure I got myself into another house of my own.

I thought about what she had said. Daphne also advised me to keep in mind that we only had one full week left to find something fast. Just hearing what she was telling me was frustrating. So, on Sunday morning, Daphne called to see if I would like to check out another house she found in Riverdale.

"Riverdale!" I said surprised. I told her that I had not really heard of Riverdale.

"I know you do not want to come to Stone Mountain where I live." She said. I told her that when we first moved to Atlanta, the brokers tried to find me a home in Stone Mountain, but I knew I wanted Christine to attend Tri-Cities High School.

Since Daphne and I did not have any more time left to look for a house, I told her that I was willing to see the house she had in mind for us in Riverdale. I saw that Riverdale was not too far from where I was living. As we pulled up to the front of the house, Christine and I said that it seemed like a very nice house. We had not even gone inside the house yet, and I told Daphne that I would take it.

"Take the house?" Daphne asked.

"Yes." I confirmed.

"Valerie, you did not even go in the house yet!" She said.

"I know." I said.

"Well, how do you know that you are going to like the house?"

"What I see on the outside already tells me that I am going to like it on the inside."

As Daphne was opening the door, Christine and I loved the house! The first thing that my little five-year-old son, Christopher said to me was, "Mommy, I love this house! This is a good house! There are no spooks in this house!" Just to hear Christopher say that took a lot of stress off of me. As we proceeded upstairs to the bedrooms, we noticed that in the master bedroom there was a bird flying around and hitting the bedroom window. Christopher said, "Mommy, this is the bird house!" He said that he was not scared to live in the bird house. I was feeling so good hearing him say those good things about the house. Daphne suggested that we go downstairs and open the front door to let the bird out. We opened the door and there was such a nice strong breeze that the bird flew right out. After all of the positive feedback that I'd received, I bought the house!

Moving Out

During the spring of 1996, my children and I were moving out of the house. When the movers came and loaded everything up, it all went smoothly for us. I had to come back the following day to do some last minute fixes on the interior of the house before the new owners moved in.

So, when I returned back, I plastered and painted and made sure that everything looked nice. After I was done there, I was very pleased to see how nice my work turned out. As Christopher, Christel and I were leaving and going down the steps to the front of the house, I noticed that the steps had started to crack one by one. I had to actually lift my children up off the steps so they would not fall.

I could not believe that was really happening to us, after we had just moved out. There was absolutely nothing wrong with those steps the day before. I immediately got my bucket of plaster. Each time I plastered, the next step would crack. I was so frustrated and was plastering as fast as I could. I knew that no one would believe what I was going through. After that, the steps looked fine. I immediately hurried Christopher and Christel into the car and we stared at the house.

"Mommy, look. The house is sad! It's crying. It doesn't want us to leave. It's sorry for the things that it's done to us!" Christopher said, pointing at the house.

"Christopher, you're right!" I said. As we continued to look at the house, we noticed that it was starting to crack straight down the middle. I said to my kids, "Forget that crap! I can't do nothing more with that house. So, let's get out of here!" I immediately pulled out of the driveway and we left!

I always heard about things like that happening to people before, but I never thought I would be the one to witness anything like it—let alone, be the one to talk about it. My children and I were finally able to get on with our lives.

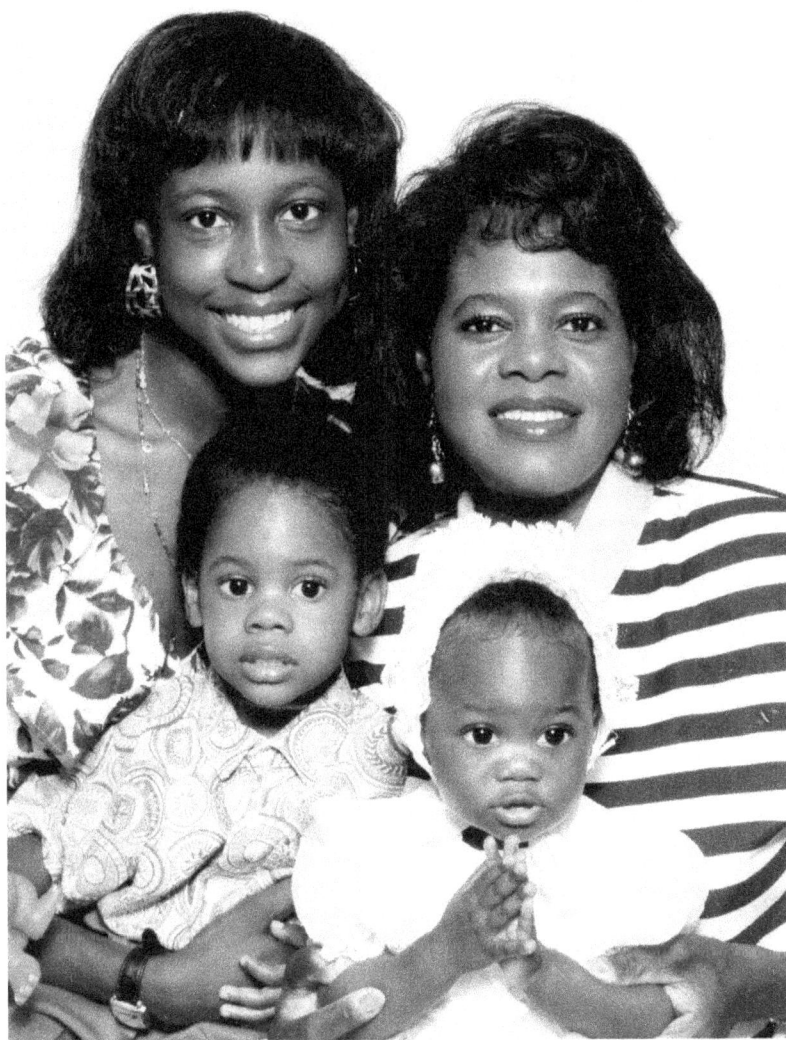

Christel Diamond Bethune's Baptism
My three children and I. Christel was wearing the same christening
outfit that my oldest daughter, Christine wore fifteen years ago.

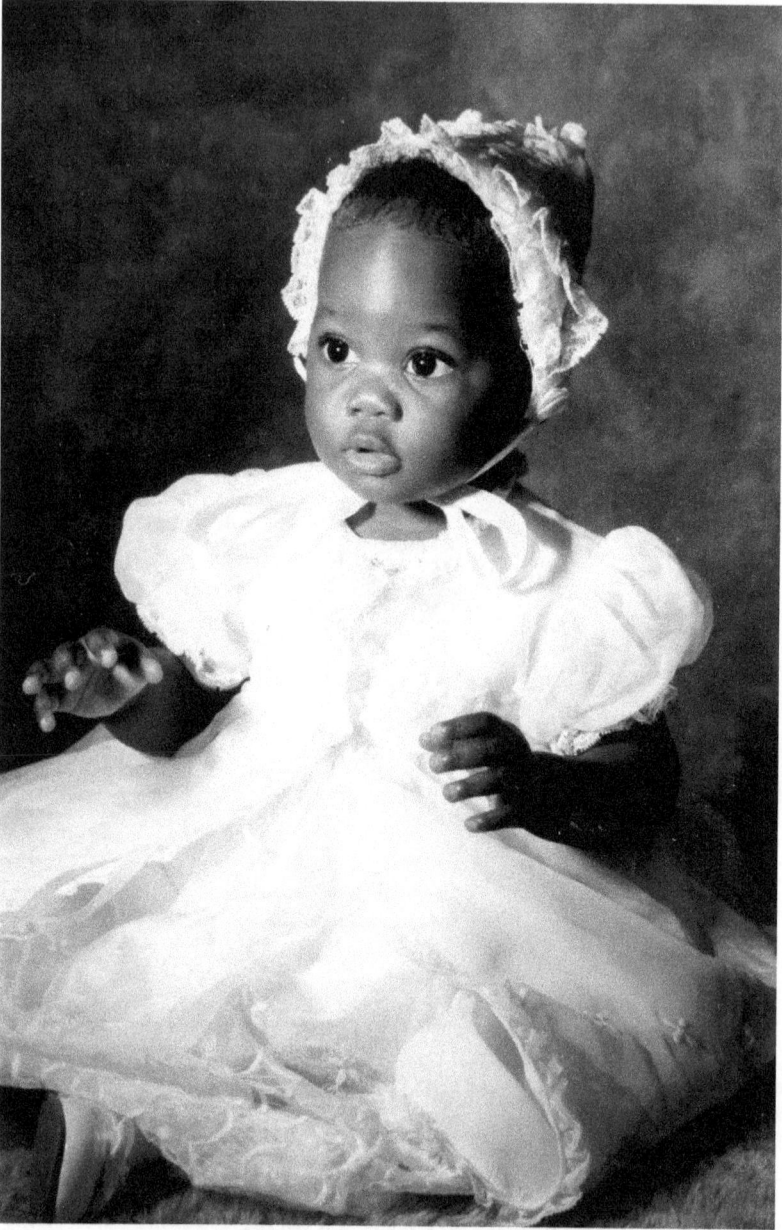

Christel Diamond Bethune's Baptism
Christel was wearing the same christening outfit that my oldest
daughter, Christine wore fifteen years ago.

CHAPTER 8

SETTLING DOWN

Yeah! We had settled down in our new home. It was a new beginning for all of us. Christopher started telling me about all of the things he had been through in our other house. In Christopher's own words, he said:

"Mommy, when I would try to go to the bathroom at night in that other house, there would be a man standing up in the hallway. He would put his hands up for me to come with him, but I would run back in my room and jump right back in my bed and wet myself." Christopher said that he was always so scared when it became nighttime. He said that he always wanted his door closed a little bit so that he would not be able to see straight down the hall at night. He also told me, "Mommy, that was why I would always run in your room and jump right in your bed, because I was so scared!" He continued to tell me that, even though the house looked very nice on the inside, to him it was still an 'ugly' house. He said that he did not like anything about that house.

I was shocked by all of the things he told me. I could not believe all that he had gone through. Just to know that, at nighttime when he had to go to bed, he always felt so scared, broke my heart. What a terrible thing for a young child to have witnessed. I told him that I was so, so sorry that he went through all of that without me even knowing anything. After hearing that, Christopher said, "Mommy, don't worry, I am not going to be scared to sleep in my room no more!" He said, "I like this house!" I was so happy and relieved to hear him say that to me.

I started thinking once again about everything we had been through, and I knew it was time to tell their father. I could not believe that Melvin was so right about that house; he said it the same day we moved in there. As I reflect back, that house did not want any of us to see anything that was going on until after he had left for good. I wanted my kids' father to know what was really going on.

Melvin's Reasons for Leaving

In Melvin's own words, he continued to tell the story about his reasons for leaving.

He said, "Boo, Boo, remember the first day when we arrived in Georgia, and I told you that I went downstairs to the basement and saw a man running to the back of the room?" He said, "When I went to look, there wasn't anybody there." I said, "Yes." He said that another time, when he went in the basement to play his guitar, the windows opened up all by themselves. Then, a voice shouted out to him saying, "Get out! Get out now! If you don't get out now, you will be sorry!" I said, "Really?" He said, "Yeah. That's when I left."

Then, he said there was yet another time when he was in the swimming pool and he could feel someone pulling him all the way down; causing him to struggle to get out. He said to me, "If you noticed, that was the reason why I never went in that swimming pool again. And remember the day when we were both trying to clean the swimming pool out and it would never get clean. Then, that very next morning when we woke up and went outside to look, it was crystal clear." I said, "Yes." He said, "It was so clean that we could not believe our eyes." I told him that I remembered that whole incident. He continued by saying, "Remember when there would always be hundreds of frogs standing around the pool?" I told him that I remembered.

He said that the last straw for him was when he was in the basement and the house told him to get out or it would kill him. He was scared out of his mind because he never in his life had anything like that happen to him before! He said that the day that he was in the driveway and about to leave, there were quarters being thrown at him. He said there was one quarter being thrown from the North, a second quarter from the South, a third quarter from the East, and a fourth quarter from the West! There were a total of four quarters being thrown at him at the exact same time! He said that he was so scared he started driving away as fast as he could to get out of there!

He kept saying to me, "Do you really think I would have left you and my kids like that?" He said that he knew from the very beginning that I would not have been able to just pick up and leave to go back to New York; he knew that I had invested too much. He said that the house told him to get out! He had just been hoping that eventually one day I would be able to see that he was telling the truth about why he had to leave.

Telling My Children's Father What I Witnessed

After hearing everything that Melvin was telling me, I started to tell him some of the things that I had witnessed. I told him that one day, I saw a giant turtle just drop to the bottom of the swimming pool and when I came back to look at it, it was gone. He said, "Wow!" I told him that another situation I encountered was when my sister and her son were visiting with us and I decided to use the microwave. The microwave had been full of ants, but nowhere else. I told him about what I had experienced with fake flowers that smelled like peppermint and dripped like blood. Melvin could not believe the things that I had gone through. I also told him that one day, when my family came down to visit with us, we all decided to go to the store and we left my father home because my foster brother was coming to see him. When we arrived back home, my father said that my foster brother, Barry had come by to visit, but the door would not open. He said that Barry waited outside for a good period of time and then just decided to go back home. But, when we came back, the door opened easily. My father was so mad because he knew that we didn't believe him. People's attitudes would also change. I told Melvin that the last thing that did it for me was when I saw that white man standing up by the steps and looking directly at me, and when I turned away from him, he was gone. I knew it was time to move out of that house for good!

I felt that the house knew how to work on each individual person that was there. I witnessed so many other things, but it was just too much to talk about. My mother told me that all of the things that I had been through could definitely be turned into a movie. She said people need to know exactly what went on.

Letter from Child Support Enforcement

When it was May 22, 1996, the Child Support Enforcement Unit informed me that there was basis for adjusting my child support order because the current order did not provide for Christine's health care needs through insurance or other means. I was so relieved to have received that information.

On June 6, 1996, my ex-husband received that new adjustment letter and he was not at all happy about it. So, on June 13, 1996, he informed the courts that he felt it was impossible for him to afford such a steep increase.

He had not been providing medical insurance for his teenage daughter and it finally caught up with him—ever since February 9, 1982, when he took Christine off of his medical insurance to put his girlfriend on.

Registering Christel into the Head Start Program

On September 3, 1996, I enrolled my youngest

daughter, Christel, into the J.F. Beaver's Clark Atlanta University's Head Start Program. Her transition to preschool was much easier than it had been for Christopher because she was able to watch her brother get up in the morning and get ready for school. Christel enjoyed preschool so much, and I noticed that she was extremely gifted in art as well.

Going to the Unemployment Office

One morning I was going to look for a job at the Unemployment Office. I was looking for work in my field, either as a secretary or a legal secretary. I was pretty much open to whatever I could find. I just wanted to work. I saw some jobs that were available, but not in my field. After finishing up on the computer, an announcement was made: "If there is anyone interested in doing cleaning work at the court buildings, please form a straight line here." I immediately went to that line.

As the interviewer was looking over my resume, he said, "You are overqualified for this cleaning position." I thought to myself, *I am so tired of always hearing that. I just want to work.* The man who was doing the hiring said to me, "I would like to offer you a supervisory position in our cleaning department. I said, "Supervisory position!" He replied with, "The position would entail being in charge of a team of employees to make sure that all the bathrooms at the various courts are thoroughly cleaned." I was a little nervous because I had never worked in that type of profession before. He assured me that, with my skills, I would do an excellent job. So, I accepted the position.

On my first day, my new boss walked over to my desk. The cleaning crew started to watch as he was dictating a letter to me. They saw that I was writing in shorthand and were so confused. I could hear people whispering and saying to each other, "How did she get this job? She was in the same line with us at the Unemployment Office for the same exact cleaning position." They were not happy about that at all. The boss started explaining to the cleaning crew that this was a contract position. He explained to them that he was their boss and I was their supervisor.

He continued stating, "We are all here to do the best job we can by making sure that all of the bathrooms are done properly. If not, you will be written up."

As time went on, we all got along nicely. Many of the employees said that they were happy that I was their supervisor because I did not pressure them and they were able to do their work well.

Court Hearings Begin

I knew that I would probably be receiving something regarding my ex-husband's objection to the increase. Sure enough, I received a letter from the court stating that: "An objection to a proposed adjusted order had been filed on this case." Our hearing was scheduled for 9:00 AM on October 15, 1996. I was really shocked that my ex-husband was doing this—especially knowing that I lived out of state. I was unable to attend the hearing at that time, but my ex-husband gave the court his response as to why he could not afford an increase.

Ex-husband's Response to the Hearing

My ex-husband said that the proposed increase that child support enforcement unit wanted to impose on him was too excessive. He said that he was currently supporting a family of four, along with child support for his daughter, Christine. He claimed that his income was responsible for the essentials like rent, food, electricity, gas, and clothing, and that he found it impossible to afford such a steep increase per month.

He further pointed out, that on October 15, 1982, we agreed on the amount that was set to be paid bi-weekly, which had always been maintained until that present time. He said that there were other stipulations that were made and never kept. He argued that the mother of his child left New York without even notifying him. That was the reason why he had requested a hearing on the matter.

My Response to the Hearing

Well, Well, Well... I remember saying to myself. I could not believe that my ex-husband had the nerve to submit that to the court knowing that none of it was even true. It was my turn to respond back. So, I sent my statement via certified mail, and I informed the court that I was unable to attend that October 15, 1996 hearing because I had two small children that were in school.

I presented to the court all of the supporting evidence

that I felt was needed to show why my ex-husband would go to many lengths just to avoid an increase in child support.

My ex-husband said that visitation rights had never been kept. How dare he say that! My ex-husband had all rights to his daughter. I attached with my statement to the court, photocopies of pictures that were taken when my ex-husband was visiting with his daughter. I thought to myself, *Why would he present this to the court knowing that it was false?*

He also said that the mother of his child left the state of New York without notifying him or the courts. This was another big shocker for me! I could not believe that my ex-husband had presented that. I attached with my statement all of the beautiful Valentine's Day cards, Mother's Day cards, Birthday cards and Christmas cards that he always sent to my residence showing the courts that he always knew where my daughter and I were living.

And finally, he said that I did not notify the court where we were living. This made no sense to me at all either. If that were true, why would the court be sending all child support monies directly to me, if they did not know where my daughter and I were living. So again, I attached to my statement letters notifying the court about when I moved; their response back to me stated that it was notated in their records.

The last thing that I pointed out in my statement was that I felt it was only fair and right that Christine's father be given an increase. I said, "This increase could greatly help with Christine's college education." I also submitted a copy of Christine's tuition statement, so that the court could see just how much we had already paid out to her school. I also addressed the fact that Christine's father should have been providing medical insurance for his daughter all of these years.

I received a letter back from the court advising me that if I did not appear on December 19, 1996 at 9:00 AM a warrant would be issued. I could not believe that this was really happening to me! I had no choice, but to appear. So, my three children and I went to New York. In the back of my mind, I was really hoping that some good would come out of all of this!

In New York City

When my children and I arrived in New York City, we were so happy to see all of our family and friends. Plus, it was close to the holidays which made it better for all of us.

On December 19, 1996, the morning of my court appearance, my girlfriend, Renee, had just gotten off from working the night shift. She was willing to drive Christine and I to court. She said that she would keep her badge on so that when she entered the building they could see right away where she works. When the hearing began, Christine and Renee patiently waited outside of the courtroom.

The hearing started promptly and my ex-husband was the first one to be given an opportunity to plead his case. I was not worried about anything because, little did he know, I had already submitted my letter with my documents attached.

After everything was being heard from my ex-husband, nothing that he presented to the court was adding up. When it was my turn to present my case, I really did not have too much to say to the court because everything that I had already said was clearly written in my statement. The only thing that I did mention was that I felt it was only fair and right that I be given an increase. I said that the increase would help with Christine's college education. After we both said what we had to say in court, they handed my letter, with all of my documents attached, over to my ex-husband for him to review. He was stunned!

He saw all of the photocopies from the cards that he was sending to Christine and I. Especially since he had claimed that I left the state of New York and he never knew where my daughter and I were living. The next thing he saw was all of the vision prescription receipts that I had already paid out for Christine, ever since she was a very young girl. Lastly, I showed copies of Christine's tuition statement that we received from the college demonstrating the amount of money we had already paid out.

After all evidence was presented to my ex-husband, he was then asked if he would like for his daughter to come into the courtroom so that he could have an opportunity to say what he does not agree with in front of her. He was so embarrassed by everything that was presented to him. He said that it was not necessary for his daughter to come in and be subjected to that and that he would do whatever he had to do for his child. I was glad that he did not want Christine to hear any of it.

One thing that came to my mind when we were both in court was, even though we were separated and then divorced, I never spoke negatively to Christine about her father or even bad mouthed him. When I would try and talk to Christine about why her father and I were not together, she was never interested to hear why. Her reply to me would always be, "You can't miss something you never had." She always said that she remembered growing up and having a great childhood. I was so grateful to hear her say that because that was something I always wanted to make sure of.

Modifying an Order of Support - 12/19/96

When I opened my mail, it was regarding the December 19, 1996 hearing. After they heard all of the proofs and testimony, my ex-husband's application was denied. So, effective December 26, 1996, I received the increase, and medical insurance for his daughter must continue. I was so happy that everything worked out well. My daughter and I no longer had to endure this and we were able to continue on with our lives.

My Boss Was Leaving

When it was the end of December, I was being approached by my boss. He said things were not going as good as it should for him. He said there were promises that were made when he took the job, but were never kept. I was not at all happy to hear that. He also told me that I probably would not be able to stay with that cleaning department because, when he leaves, they would be bringing in their own crew. I thought about everything he had said. At that time, I felt that I did not have too much to lose and would just try it out and see what happens.

Soon after my boss left, it became clear that he was right about everything. They did bring in their own people and I was not able to work under those conditions. Therefore, I had no choice but to resign.

Summer of 1998 – Kids Fest Coloring Contest

My little daughter, Christel, was doing so well with her colors. So, during August of 1998, Publix Supermarket had a Kids Fest Coloring Contest that was held at the store where we lived. I signed Christel up to compete with the other children. The store's cutoff age for participating in that contest was twelve years old, but at the time Christel was only five years old.

After entering, Christel was contacted via telephone that she had been chosen as the winner of the 1998 Kids Fest Coloring Contest. The store wanted Christel to come in and take pictures with the manager and claim her prize. I was so happy and proud of her!

Going to a Movie Shoot

During September 1998, when I was forty-six years old, my oldest daughter, Christine, was consistently pursuing her acting career. Her movie shoot took place in Senoia,

Georgia. The movie was called "Mama Flora's Family." They were also in need of some extras to appear in that movie. So, Christine decided that when we got there, we should also try out for a part.

When we arrived in Senoia, Georgia at 11:30 AM, they had all varieties of food that were constantly being prepared for everyone throughout the course of the day. The casting crew of the movie saw that I had two young children, ages seven and five. They were so glad that my kids could participate in that movie as well as myself because they were in need of some more children.

Firstly, Christopher and Christel were escorted to be fitted for the clothes they would be wearing. I had to go in a totally different area. When I saw Christopher and Christel, I thought they looked so cute, but the look on Christel's face was not at all happy.

She did not like the way they fixed her hair for the movie. She had two long loose braided pig tails sticking out, with long ribbons hanging from the tips of the braids. Christel knew that I never fix her hair like that and she could not understand why they did that to her hair. They fixed her hair according to the era the movie took place in, but Christel was too young to understand any of that. She felt that she looked ugly.

Secondly, she did not appreciate wearing the long brown dress with the leather boots that they gave her. She said the boots were too tight, too hard, and her feet were hurting. So, they gave her a second pair of boots. She complained that those leather boots were too big and too hard as well. They had no other boots to give her. They felt it was better for the boots to be slightly bigger than to be too tight; there were no more boots her size.

Thirdly, Chistopher and Christel had a scene where they had to run, and Christopher tried his best by holding her hand so that she could run with him. Christine stayed by their side during that scene which she was also in. Christel was not having it and was tired of running. Around 4:00 PM the crew decided to give Christel some jello. After eating the jello, she was so happy. The crew was so amazed and could not believe it. After that, Christel continued her scene without anymore problems.

Shooting for the movie was over at 7:00 PM for all of us, but Christine had many more takes to do. Christopher and Christel had a long day and were tired, so we slept in the car overnight until Christine was finished. We all had a very nice day and night—except for Christel.

Christel Happy to Use Her Prize

When the summer was over and Christel's birthday was approaching, it was time for her to use the prize she had won from the Kids Fest Coloring Contest. That prize certificate entitled her to receive: (1) free bag of Publix 14 oz. potato chips, (1) free package of Publix chocolate chip cookies, (4) free bottles of Publix 2 liter soft drinks, (1) free half gallon of Publix ice cream, and (1) free 1/4 sheet cake of her choice from the Publix Bakery. She was so happy when we picked up her cake for her Saturday birthday—on October 24, 1998. She had a black ballerina on her yellow cake with butter cream icing that consisted of beautiful roses and fresh strawberries, which she loved. She also wanted her cake to say "Happy Birthday Christel." That was a very nice sixth birthday celebration to remember!

School Positions

When it was February 1999, I decided to inquire at the school where my children attended to see if there were any openings at their after school enrichment program. I already knew some of the people that were working there. My friend, Valerie, was the one who told me to inquire since she had just started working there. So, I did.

The school got back to me and wanted to hire me. They discussed my many interests and decided that I would teach art to the students. As time went on, the school was so impressed with what the children were grasping, that they wanted me to expand in other areas, as well.

During the month of May 3, 1999, I decided to take on a full-time position at another school as a para-professional. I completed all of my training and began working in the Kindergarten classroom. Since, I was holding down two Public School positions, I had to enroll Christopher and Christel in the before school program for breakfast in the mornings and in the after school enrichment program in the afternoons.

Then, in the evening hours when Christine got off work, I would drive to the train station to pick her up. Needless to say, this was a very busy and challenging schedule for all of us because I had to get everyone to their destinations on time in order for me to get myself back to the school where I was working by 7:30 AM.

Problems Arise

After working as a para-professional full-time, I decided I no longer wanted to work there and put any more stress on myself to stay. Therefore, I decided to resign.

I continued on with the after school enrichment program at my children's school in the afternoons. But, at least they did not have to get up extra, extra early in the mornings for school anymore. So, everything worked out well for us.

Summer Program

When school was almost over, they were offering a summer program at my children's school. I decided it would be enjoyable for them to be with children their own age. Therefore, I applied and was hired to work there for the summer.

Court Hearings Were Over

My ex-husband alerted me in advance that I would be receiving a letter from the court, now that Christine had reached the age of twenty-one. On a good note, my ex-husband no longer had any outstanding payments for his daughter. He wanted me to make sure that I informed the court that all monies from him were paid in full.

On June 8, 1999, I received a letter that I had to appear before the court on August 2, 1999, at 9:15 AM. Since I was unable to attend that hearing, I submitted my letter on July 22, 1999.

Ex-husband's Final Child Support Hearing - 8/2/99

My letter was submitted at the August 2, 1999, hearing. The court's findings were that the arrears should be adjusted, the order of support should be terminated, and that my ex-husband was no longer responsible for child support enforcement services.

My ex-husband signed the verification letter that I submitted and it was given to him in court. He signed, confirming that he had read the contents of my letter and believed it to be true. Those years of child support payments from Christine's father were finally over and he was happy.

Christine's father told me time and time again that his life started going bad for him the day my father went with him to purchase his red Monte Carlo car. He said that, deep down inside, he was young, not ready, and that was when he started "hanging out." He said that he never wanted a divorce, but he knew why I did what I had to do.

After School Program Has Ended

The after school program at my children's school ended during September 1999. I appreciated the opportunity to work there. I decided to pursue other options that would allow me the flexibility and availability for my three children. My oldest daughter was very busy pursuing her acting career, and I wanted to make sure that I was available for her.

I was certified to work as a family day care provider. After exploring that option, my children all loved the availability that came with me being at home when they need me.

Halloween Coloring Contest at Publix

After Christel had won the Kids Fest Coloring Contest previously, the store was having a Halloween Coloring Contest. Christopher was always a very competitive person and was not going to miss out on that contest. So, he also entered. Christopher was eight years old and Christel was seven years old. They both won! Between the two of them, they received Crayon fun packs and coupons consisting of: four boxes of 12 oz. Pepsi sodas and four big bags of Doritos of their choice. After that, there was no stopping them, and I knew their artistic talents were only going to get better and better.

Kids Coloring Contest at Publix

During December 1999, Publix had another Kids Coloring Contest that Christel wanted to enter. Christel continued winning contests. After she found out that she won, pictures were taken at the store and she recieved a prize. Christel was so happy. Thanks to Publix for having contests like that!

A Review of Child Support for My Two Youngest Children

During November 6, 2000, it was time for my child support case to be reviewed for modification for my two youngest children. The money that I was receiving from their father per week was just not enough. I decided that all monies should be payable through the child support collection unit, so that they could keep track of everything that he sends. On December 14, 2000, it was ordered. On March 3, 2001, papers were filed in court. Months went by. Then, on September 25, 2001, I informed the court that I would be testifying via telephone. My papers regarding my financial disclosure affidavit were forwarded and my out of state petition was filed. My telephonic hearing was scheduled for October 25, 2001.

I showed the court that, despite how well my children were being cared for, I needed the additional financial help. So, for the October 25, 2001, hearing I sent documents to the court showing what an excellent job both Christopher—who was in the fourth grade at the time—and Christel—who was in the second grade at the time—were doing in school. I sent a copy of a picture of each of them so that the court could see exactly what they looked like. I also sent photocopies of their report cards that they received from school, as well as their teacher's comments.

I had the telephonic hearing that was scheduled on October 25, 2001, but the court had to issue another telephonic hearing because their father was not prepared. That hearing was then scheduled for December 6, 2001, between the hours of 10:00 AM and 1:00 PM. That meant that I had to be available between those hours.

We did have that hearing, but their father still did not have the documentation that the court needed.

A Telephonic Hearing

At 3:00 PM on January 24, 2002, my two youngest children's father and I were both sworn in at that telephonic hearing.

After everything that I had gone through by testifying and providing all of my documentation, he still failed to present any of his documentation with an adequate explanation. He told the court that he did not want an adjournment to bring in his documentation, but that he earns a substantial amount of money as a construction worker. Therefore, the hearing was over and I was told that I would be receiving a letter stating the court's findings.

I received the court's letter informing me that the petition was granted and it became effective February 15, 2002. I was thankful for what the court had done.

Being Involved at School

I always made it a point to be extremely involved in the curriculum that was given at my children's school. I encouraged the teachers to keep me informed as to how my children were doing. I made it a point to attend their meetings, be heavily involved in my children's activities, as well as volunteer whenever I could.

On April 27, 2004, the school presented me with a Certificate of Appreciation in recognition of my support, involvement, and contributions to the REACH program as a Volunteer, Mentor, and Partner in Education.

Working in Retail

During the month of November 2005, my health was doing very well. I started working at the Home Depot store that had just opened up near my home. I worked as a kitchen and bath design consultant for about six months. I really enjoyed what I was doing—especially interacting with the customers. The only problem was, since the store was still very new, we were constantly being sent home due to a lack of customers coming into the store. I would walk in, be told it was going to be slow, and then be instructed to go right back home. As a single parent, I could no longer continue to keep that up. Therefore, I had no choice but to resign.

Marketing and Research

I decided to make some new changes in my life. I branched out into a whole different type of career. I decided to go into the field of Marketing and Research as an independent contractor. I had all the skills needed to do that type of job, and my children loved what I was doing.

Christine Touring with The Lion King - 7/5/06

On July 5, 2006, right after the big July 4th holiday, my daughter left to tour with *The Lion King.*

That tour was the opportunity of a lifetime for her! She was able to travel all over the world. I missed her dearly. She was away for such a long period of time. When her schedule permitted her to do so, she was able to fly home. *The Lion King* tour was one of her most memorable journeys.

Part-Time Position - Working for Outbound Collections

September 5, 2006, I started working for Outbound Collections. It was a temporary, part-time, seasonal assignment. I kept accurate accounts of the customer's payments and helped resolve complaints as they arised.

Being Seen by a Private Doctor for Lupus

I was seeing a private doctor on my own for my lupus due to a lack of health insurance. It was definitely not working out for me at all. I really needed to be in a hospital setting where I would be able to receive full treatment.

Lupus Flare-up – 1/16/07

On January 16, 2007, I had a doctor's appointment. I was having a lupus flare-up. The doctor started me on Prednisone because my hair was falling out terribly. For example, I would take six 5 mg pills for three days, then five 5 mg pills for three days, then four 5 mg pills for three days, then three 5 mg pills for three days, then two 5 mg pills for three days, and finally, one 5 mg pill daily.

Last Day of Work

My temporary position with Outbound Collections had ended. My last day was February 9, 2007. I really enjoyed working there and meeting new people.

My Doctors Appointment

On March 22, 2007, I had a doctors appointment. My weight was 191 pounds due to being on so much Prednisone. Also, the high blood pressure medicine that I was taking, called Sular, did not agree with me. Therefore, my doctor decided that I should stop taking it. I was still taking my 25 mg Hydrochlorothiazide water pill. My potassium level at the time was very low, so I had to take Klor Con once a day, for ten days. At that time, I was off all Prednisone medication.

Seeking A New Venture

After seeing my doctor and getting my health back on track, I decided to seek a new venture. I wanted to become a foster parent. I figured that since I had two young teenagers living at home with me, why not take on some other young teens that we would enjoy having in our home. My children and I were all in agreement.

Children's Father Was Extremely Ill

On April 24, 2007, I received a letter from the court stating that I was summoned to appear before the court on June 21, 2007, at 9:30 AM. My two youngest children's father, Melvin, had a change of circumstances. He had three strokes and was requesting that he be given a downward modification of child support that was already entered from January 24, 2002. Since, I was living out of state I had to testify in court via telephone.

Temporary Modification of Support

We had the telephonic hearing on June 21, 2007. The court granted Melvin a temporary reduction of his child support monies based on the letter that he presented from his doctor, dated June 11, 2007. His payments commenced on July 1, 2007 through the support collection unit.

Presenting Character Evidence to the Court

After that hearing was over, I was going to have yet another hearing. So, on August 15, 2007, I was happy to share with the court via letter, once again, my children's grades in school and how nicely they have both grown.

The pictures that I sent to the court showed that Christopher was sixteen years old, attending high school, and was planning to major in Engineering/Technology. Christel's picture showed that she was fourteen years old and that she had graduated from the eighth grade, and would soon be attending the same high school as her brother. Her intention was to major in Cosmetology. I stated that their grades had been exceptional.

I also shared that, "Yes, my life has been a great struggle as a single parent, but I made the decision to give my children a better way of life." I noted to the court that I was still driving my same car that I had purchased new while living in New York City.

Everything that was presented to the court on my behalf was reviewed. On August 28, 2007, at 1:45 PM, I testified via telephone. After the court heard all of the proofs of both testimonies, the only evidence that my children's father was able to present was the same June 11th letter from his doctor. He did not produce any updated medical records indicating that he was still unable to work. So, on September 7, 2007, the court said that the original order for the same amount he was paying would be automatically reinstated without prejudice to Petitioner's right to re-file.

Collecting Disability

After going through that hearing on August 28, 2007, Melvin informed me that he was now collecting disability. He advised me to go to the social security office and apply for disability for his two children.

On September 7, 2007, I did just that and a decision was made on our claim. We received a letter back from social security on September 14, 2007 stating that my children were entitled to monthly benefits all the way back from February of 2007 and would continue thereon.

My children's father contacted us via telephone and wanted to know if his children were receiving their benefits. I told him they were.

His Comments Regarding Disability

Melvin was happy that they were receiving their benefits. He mentioned to me on the telephone that he couldn't believe this was happening to him. He said, "I always loved to work. If I am not able to work, I will be so bored because that's what keeps me happy."

My children's father was not the type of person who would just want to lie around the house with nothing to do. He always had to keep himself busy doing something. I knew exactly what he meant.

As he continued talking, he told me to please do not take what he said to me personally. He told me that since I was receiving his disability money from his illness, maybe that could be a way for him to at least help us out some more. I told him that it really did help us out a lot. He continued saying that he never had to worry about his kids. He told me that I have been doing such an excellent job with them, and I deserve the money that I got for them. I told him that I definitely understood everything he was saying. No matter what was going on, my children's father said that he still remained hopeful that maybe one day he would be able to return back to work again.

Totally Disabled

On November 28, 2007, I received word from my children's father that he was totally disabled due to having three strokes, severe high blood pressure, and other related medical conditions.

Petition for Modification

I received a letter from the court for a petition for modification of an order. I was summoned to appear before the court on January 3, 2008, at 9:15 AM. Their father requested a reduction in child support benefits to be commensurate with his disability income. I testified via telephone. Child support was awarded to him at a smaller amount per week, effective January 4, 2008, and retroactive to November 27, 2007. That small amount of child support monies was fine for me because his children were still receiving the social security benefits. I had gone through so much in order for my two youngest children to be able to get what was only fair and right for them. Some people would have definitely given up. I thank God each and every day for the knowledge I had been given. I kept striving for more no matter what and had an excellent outcome through it all.

Working With Young Children/Teens

After completing all of my foster care training classes, I reached out to the different agencies and was thoroughly approved. I was happy to have been given the opportunity to work with young children as well as teens.

When they were in my care, I registered the children in school. I attended school meetings and programs as needed. I worked closely with their case managers and shared information towards the children's progress and their goals. I arranged recreational activities, as well as the cultural and spiritual needs of the children, as it prepared them to be self-sufficient and responsible. I had a wonderful and exciting year with them! On May 31, 2008, I received a Certificate of Appreciation for outstanding service as a foster parent.

Admitted to Piedmont Hospital – 3/2009

I became extremely ill and was admitted to Piedmont Hospital during March 2009.

Lymph Node Biopsy

On March 16, 2009, when I was fifty-six years old, I became so ill that my thirty-one-year-old daughter, Christine, had no choice but to rush me to Emergency at Piedmont Hospital. I was admitted to Piedmont Hospital at 10:27 AM due to painfully swollen lymph nodes on the right side of my neck, chills and fever, diarrhea, nausea, and vomiting.

A biopsy was done on my lymph nodes and it turned out to be negative. They kept me in the hospital an extra week so that more tests could be administered and to make sure that nothing else developed. I thought it could have been my lupus flaring up, but it still was hard for them to diagnose.

My daughter, Christine, knew that I would not have gone to the hospital on my own due to my lack of medical insurance. On March 23, 2009, I was discharged from the hospital and was given a discharge medication report. I was told to continue taking the Extra Strength Tylenol at 1000 mg every six hours as needed for fever. I was instructed to continue taking Atenolol for my high blood pressure at 25 mgs once daily, orally. I was also given a new medication that I needed to continue. It was called Metoclopramide (Reglan) at 5 mgs. I took that four times a day orally as needed for nausea (before meals and at bedtime).

Since my blood pressure was not high during the time I was in the hospital, I was told to stop taking Hydrochlorothiazide at 25 mgs. I was also told to stop taking the Ibuprophen capsule (Motrin 1B) 400 mg that I was taking every four hours. After my 5 mg Prednisone pill was tapered off and finished, I no longer had to take it.

The Teacher Who Made a Difference in My Son, Christopher's Life

Christopher's art teacher, Ms Spivey was that one special teacher who made a difference in his life. When Christopher entered Riverdale High School, he decided that he only wanted to major in Engineering and Technology. But, when it came to his third year of high school, he took Ms. Spivey's art class and that changed everything for him. Ms. Spivey brought out all of the artistic talents that he possessed. He was chosen to compete in the 7th Annual 13th Congressional District High School Art Competition.

During the time of my son's competition, I was so, so sick. My lupus was flaring up so badly, but I tried to make the best of each moment of that day. Christopher was awarded a Certificate of Achievement for Outstanding Achievement in Fundamentals of Design.

During his last year of high school, he was totally dedicated to the idea of changing his career plans. He was so excited by the idea of majoring in art that he decided that when he graduated, he would immediately attend college during the summer months at The Art Institue of Atlanta and not wait until the fall semester.

Christopher Was Graduating

After being in the hospital in March, I did not know what to expect. My life had so many twists and turns from being so sick.

On Saturday, May 30, 2009, I was so happy to be at the Georgia Dome celebrating the morning of my son's high school graduation. Christopher's commencement exercises began at 9:00 AM. It was such a beautiful day, and I was so proud of all his accomplishments.

Getting Extremely Sick – 11/2009

During the month of November 2009, I was getting really sick again. It felt like my whole entire body was burning up and I was on fire. I literally felt like I was burning alive. The skin on my back was so raw that it was coming right off of my body. At that time, I did not even go to the hospital. I went to a private doctor in my area because I did not have any medical insurance. The doctor prescribed a Silver Sulfadiazine (1%) cream. He said that if there was no change, to please make sure I get to a hospital immediately! After using that cream, it started giving me some relief, but what I was going through was definitely not normal at all. I still needed help!

Lupus Flare-up-Admitted to Grady Memorial Hospital – 12/16/09

On December 16, 2009, I was admitted to Grady Memorial Hospital. I was glad that I was there so that I could be monitored more closely.

On December 19, 2009, my diagnosis showed a lupus flare-up with very severe rashes all over—my arms, chest, and back which were absolutely raw. The doctors were trying to figure out what was causing all of this. I was also given a flu shot in my right arm and a pneumonia shot in my left arm. Both tests came back negative, but they found protein in my urine. On December 21, 2009, I was discharged from the hospital. When I returned back home, I made sure that I checked my blood pressure daily. After going through that terrible episode, I looked forward to a better year ahead.

Referred to the Renal Clinic

In the New Year of 2010, when I was fifty-seven years old, the doctors were still trying to see what was really going on with my lupus. So, on January 26, 2010, I went to Grady Memorial Hospital to have some lab work done because the doctors were still not clear of my diagnosis and what must be done. After they saw my lab results, I was informed that my kidneys were involved and I was referred to the Renal Clinic for a proper diagnosis.

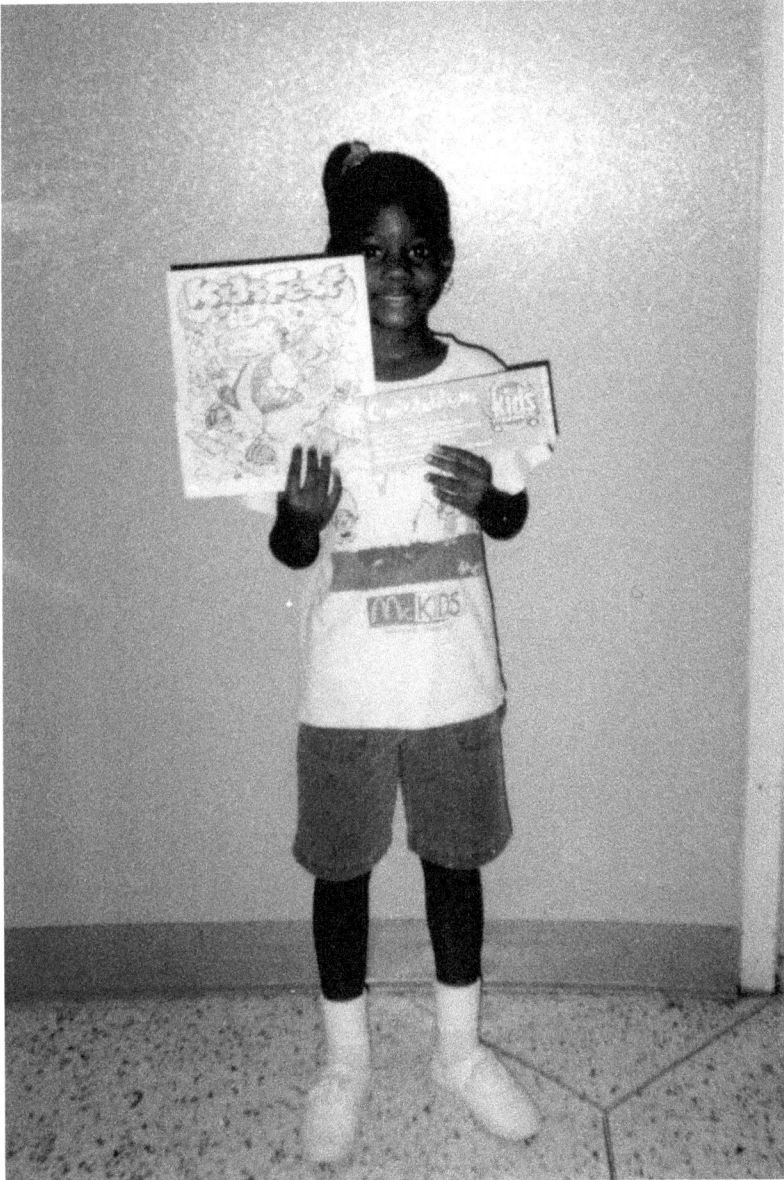

My daughter, Christel won the Kids Fest Coloring Contest at five years old. Picture was taken at Publix during August 1998.

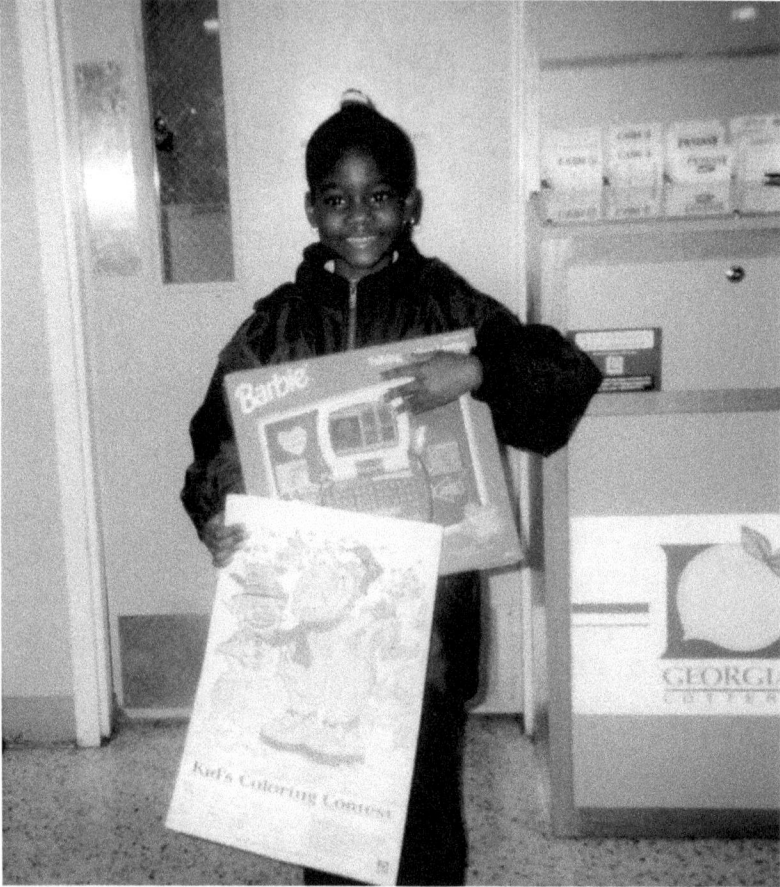

My daughter, Christel won the Kids Fest Coloring Contest. Picture was taken at Publix during December 1999. She was seven years old.

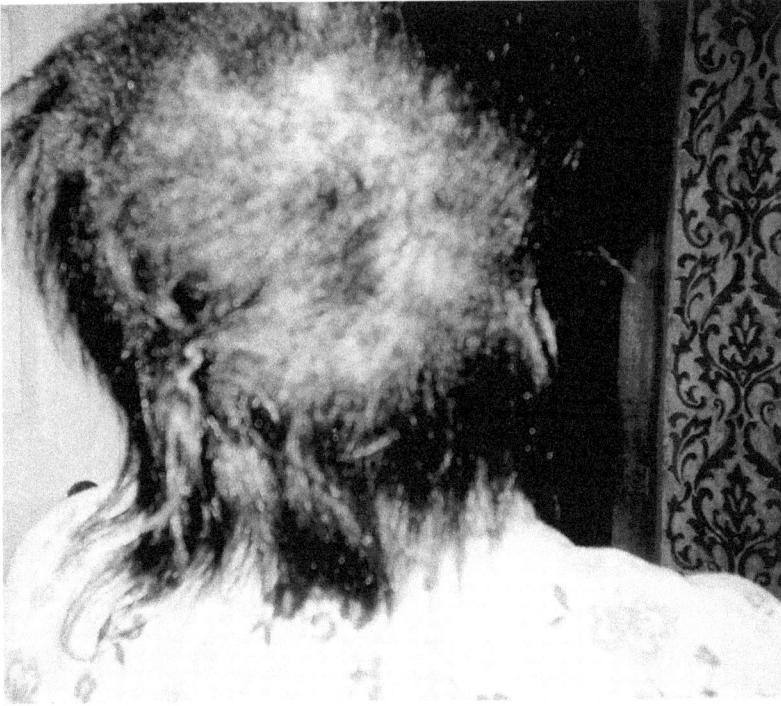

Lupus Flare-up: My hair was falling out terribly.

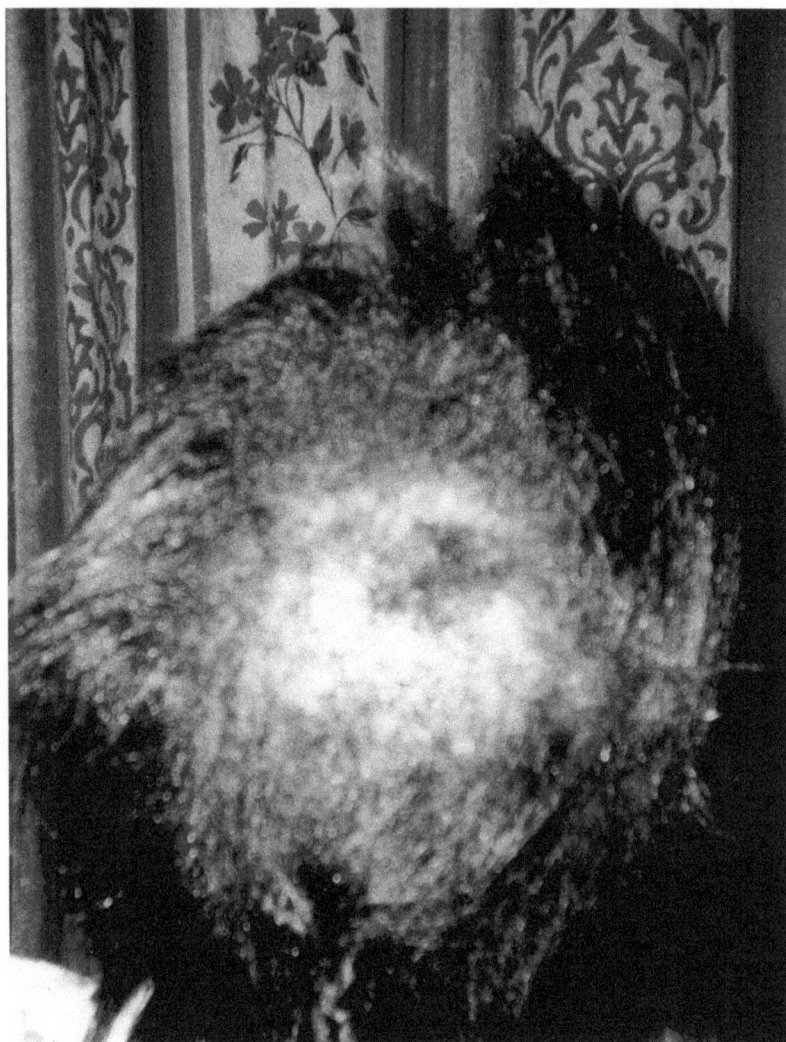

Lupus Flare-up: I continued losing hair.

CHAPTER 9

OVERCOMING OBSTACLES

The morning of February 24, 2010, at 11:50 AM, I was at the Renal Clinic. I sat down with my doctor so that he could explain everything to me. He informed me that all of my lab results came back and showed that I have Lupus Nephritis. The Renal Clinic issued a radiology order form for a kidney biopsy to be done. They needed to find out exactly what stage my kidneys were in.

Kidney Biopsy

On March 12, 2010, I was admitted to Grady Memorial Hospital for the renal and left kidney biopsy to be done. My mother and sister, Vanessa, rushed down from New York to be with me. Before going to the hospital, my feet were swollen so badly that I had to buy a pair of men's extra wide slippers. My entire body was swelling up with fluid. My mother was trying to assure me that whatever the doctors were going to have to do, I should try not to worry. She said, "With today's technology, the procedure should go okay and not like it was when you were younger." I appreciated my family being there by my side. Their support was what I really needed.

I began thinking to myself how horrible it was to be in this condition and feeling so helpless. I could not even stand up on my own two feet; I was totally bedridden. Thank goodness for my children; they were always there to help me.

That was the most horrible thing I have ever had to experience. At that time, I did not have any type of strength or energy. I could not even stand up without assistance. And as far as cooking was concerned, that was out of the question for me. My hands were so badly swollen that I was too weak to touch anything. My children had to assist me with everything.

After the biopsy, I was told to monitor my urine for any signs of blood, as well as the site where the biopsy had been done. They had me on a 2-gram low sodium diet, which was not a problem for me since I do not add extra salt in my diet. I was told that activities can be done as tolerated. I was discharged on March 13, 2010.

While my mother and sister, Vanessa, were visiting with us, Christopher and Christel carefully watched how my sister was preparing everything for me. That way, when their aunt leaves, they would be able to continue to keep everything under control. I was so grateful for everything she did.

Admitted Back to Grady Memorial Hospital on 3/23/10

Oh no! It was March 23, 2010, only ten days later, when I was admitted back to Grady Memorial Hospital after my kidney biopsy procedure had been done. Christine was living in California, pursuing her acting career. She decided to pick up and come back to Atlanta while I was totally out of sorts with my kidneys. My girlfriend and my daughter's friends transported me back and forth to my doctor's appointments. I appreciated everything that they were doing for me.

Now that I had already been informed that I had Lupus Nephritis, the doctors put me on numerous types of medications while I was in the hospital. The swelling throughout my body and the severe high blood pressure I was experiencing, knocked my system way out of control. I knew what I was going through was not going to be an easy fix. The doctors told me not to worry, that I would be okay. They said, "In time, things will go back to normal." They continued to encourage me to be patient because they said, "All of this did not happen overnight." I was also given a renal diet pamphlet to keep. To sustain this was not going to be a problem for me because I actually really liked this diet.

I could not believe the amount of medications that I was given! It showed just how bad my health had become. The medications that I had to take were:

Amlodipine one 10 mg tablet (to treat high blood pressure), Bumetanide one 1 mg tablet (strong water pill), Clonidine 0.3 mg tablet, then I was reduced to Clonidine 0.2 mg tablet, then I was reduced to Clonidine 0.1 mg tablet (Clonidine was used with my other medications to also treat high blood pressure). I also had to take Ergocalciferol Capsules at 50,000 (I was Vitamin D deficient) Esomeprazole 40 mg (1) Cap (it was used for acid reflux), Fenofibrate 160 mg tablet (it helped control levels of blood fats and lower bad cholesterol), Furosemide 20 mg tablet (water pill), Hydrochlorothiazide 25 mg tablet (water pill), Lisinopril 5 mg tablet, and then I was on a 40 mg tablet of Lisinopril (to treat high blood pressure), Metolazone 5 mg tablet (water pill), Metoprolol XL 25 mg tablet (to treat high blood pressure), Metoprolol Tartrate 50 mg tablets (to treat high blood pressure), Mycophenolate 500 mg tablet (for the kidneys), Potassium 10 meq CR tab (to treat low amounts of potassium in the blood), Potassium Chloride Extended-Release tabs (treating low potassium blood levels), Potassium Chloride Oral Liquid (treating low potassium blood levels), Prednisone 10 mg tablet, then increased to 20 mgs for my lupus, Promethazine 25 mg tablet (for nausea), and Triamcinolone 0.1% Cream for skin, but not on face, and Triamcinolone 0.1% Ointment (reduce itching of the skin).

It had been a long haul for me at Grady. I was discharged on March 31, 2010, along with the hospital's very nice renal diet pamphlet that I was given during my stay. Since my blood pressure was extremely high, and changed from hour to hour, I had to make sure that it was monitored daily and that I was taking my medications as instructed. I continued my activities as tolerated and tried not to exert myself too much. My family always told me that I was doing too much and to slow down—I took their advice.

My Mother Came to Atlanta to Be With Me

My mother, who was eighty-nine years old, knew the condition that I was in and wanted to come to Atlanta to be with me no matter what. My sister, Vanessa, was not at all pleased that she was traveling that long distance from New York to Atlanta by Amtrak all by herself. But, my mother was determined to come. After arriving from that long commute, my mother came in my room and sat down at the desk. Her head was going down as I was talking to her. When I came over and lifted her head up, her eyes were rolling back. I kept calling out to her, but she did not respond. I immediately called my son to come in my room. We immediately called an ambulance. Just before they arrived, my mom woke up. The paramedics thoroughly checked her, but felt that due to her age they had to use certain precautions and took her to the nearest hospital.

She was admitted into the hospital on April 13, 2010 and was not at all happy to be there. They carefully monitored her. On April 16, 2010, they discharged her. She was given a prescription for Hydralazine 50 mg tablet for high blood pressure. After returning back to my house, all of the family felt it would be better for her to get back home immediately. Plus, since she was feeling much better, we did not want her to take any medications without her own doctor approving it. After that, we never wanted her to take a long trip like that ever again. The only trip safe enough should be by plane, and not by herself.

My mother felt so bad about what had happened. It was the anxiety of coming to Atlanta that did it for her. She said, "I came to take care of you, and you wound up taking care of me." I told her that was definitely okay, and I was so glad that she was feeling much better.

Renal Clinic Appointments

On April 27, 2010, I had a followup doctors appointment at 1:50 PM at the Renal Clinic at Grady. Time had passed since I last saw my doctor, and I had learned a lot more about Lupus Nephritis and how to cope. I was on the following medications: Amlodipine 10 mg, Bumex 1 mg, Ergocalciferol 50,000, KDur 10 meq, Lisinopril 40 mg, Metoprolol 50 mg, and Prednisone 10 mg.

I was a little nervous when I was sitting at the doctor's office. My doctor explained everything to me. He was the same doctor who took care of me every step of the way when I was admitted to Grady Memorial Hospital in April.

As we looked at the chart on the wall in his office, he explained to me the different stages that our kidneys can go through. He informed me that, from all the tests that I had taken, my kidneys were at Stage III and I must get my body back under control. We were in another New Year. On January 18, 2011, I was taking the following medications for Lupus Nephritis:

Amlodipine 10 mg one tablet daily, Bumetanide 1 mg

one tablet twice a day, Lisinopril 40 mg one tablet daily, Potassium 10 MEQ CR two tablets daily, Prednisone 5 mg tablet (one 5 mg tablet and break the other tablet in half = 1½ tablets every morning), Metoprolol 50 mg two tablets every morning, and one tablet every evening, Mycophenolate (Cellcept) a 500 mg tablet to be taken three times a day.

After a few months went by, we were in the month of May and my health seemed to finally be getting better and better.

Giving Back

I always enjoyed giving back whenever I could. So, I decided to work with one of the charities where I lived. The work I was doing for them was very, very detail-oriented and demanded a lot of my attention. The best part about the job was that I was able to work from home.

The Teachers Who Made a Difference in My Daughter, Christel's Life

Christel's Cosmetology teacher, Mrs. Harris, at River-dale High School was an excellent teacher who made a difference in my daughter's life. Christel always looked forward to going to her cosmetology class. Mrs. Harris always extended herself to my daughter when she needed extra help. She knew that Christel was interested in becoming a Master Cosmetologist. Christel was always so grateful to have such a caring and thoughtful teacher.

Another teacher who made a difference in my

daughter's life was Ms. Spivey. Ms. Spivey was the same art teacher that my son had. When I enrolled Christel in Ms. Spivey's sculpting class, all of her artistic talents came out. I was able to see just how great of a sculptor she really was. Ms Spivey was also amazed at Christel's artistic capabilities. Ms. Spivey would tell me that, when she would ask the class to sculpt something, she did not have to worry about Christel because she knew that whatever Christel sculpted, it would be "way over the top." Ms. Spivey said that Christel's art was always so outstanding that she awarded Christel with the Outstanding Artist Award. After seeing all of what Christel was capable of doing, I told Christel, "If you can sculpt, that means you can definitely do nails, as well."

Christel Has Graduated

On Tuesday, May 24, 2011, my youngest daughter, Christel, graduated from Riverdale High School. Her graduation ceremony took place at 3:00 PM at the Georgia Dome. My family and I were all in attendance. It was such a good feeling knowing that my youngest child had now graduated. I was so proud of all of my daughter's accomplishments and looked forward to great things ahead for her.

I encouraged Christel to start studying so that she would be able to get her Master Cosmetology license. There were two parts to the test that she had to take: the written examination and the practical examination.

The more she studied, the more I quizzed her. I knew she was ready to take the exam. On January 19, 2012,

Christel took the written exam and passed! I was so proud of her for taking that first step and accomplishing that. The next part of the test would be the practical examination, which would be all hands on. She looked forward to taking that next test, but she still had plenty of time to prepare herself.

Doctors Appointments - Do I have Gout?

The years had just been flying by. During February of 2012, I was seen at the Rheumatology Clinic at Grady Memorial Hospital. As I was sitting down in the room, I showed my doctor my left ring finger. I had noticed little lumps on the sides of my finger that were starting to develop more around the knuckles, but I had not experienced any pain. The doctor said that it looked a little like gout. I said, "Gout! How did I develop gout?" I was told to watch and see how my fingers looked when I saw the doctor at my next appointment at the Lupus Clinic. Other than that, everything seemed to be going okay.

I began thinking to myself, *I have been so near death with all that I have been going through.* I felt so blessed to have seen the age of sixty years old. God pulled me through, even when I did not know from day to day if I would even make it! My own life experiences have been amazing!

During the month of July 2012, I did have a doctors appointment, but due to unforeseen commitments that month, I was unable to see my doctor. My finger was still swelling up and getting bigger and bigger around the knuckles. When I touched it, it was very painful. It felt like it was on fire. I was taking Ibuprofen tablets every four hours for the pain and swelling. I also started taking three tablespoons of black cherry juice that I purchased from the pharmacy, just in case it was gout. The pharmacy told me not to eat any junk food (cakes, cookies, pies, etc.). I was already taking things to relieve the pain in my finger, but still nothing helped. So, on September 11, 2012, I was hoping to find the answers that I needed.

It was the morning of September 11, 2012. My left ring finger was still swollen and nothing had changed. I looked forward to hearing what the doctors were going to say about all of this during my clinic visit. During that time, I was on two 5 mg Prednisone tablets daily, one 25 mg tablet of hydrochlorothiazide, one Lisinopril 40 mg tablet (as needed) for blood pressure, one Bumetanide 1 mg tablet (as needed for swelling), and four 500 mg tablets of Mycophenolate (Cellcept).

Although I was going through some problems with my health, I did not let it get me down. I still smiled and reminisced about my life in general. I felt so good inside, but I do not know why. I just felt like it was going to be a beautiful day for whatever reason.

When Christopher, Christel and I arrived at the clinic at 11:00 AM, I could not believe how empty the clinic was that morning. I had to ask the receptionists, "Where is everybody today?" They replied, "A lot of people cancelled their appointments today."

When my children and I were just about to sit down in the clinic waiting room area, I was informed that there was a lupus support group meeting that was held a little earlier that morning. The ladies informed me about what had taken place: They said that there was a very young teenage girl that came with her family and that they had just found out that their daughter had lupus. At that meeting, they said that everyone shared with the family their ideas, stories, and tips for about an hour.

After hearing what the ladies were telling me, I told them that I also had lupus when I was very young, so I definitely understood what that family was going through. We continued to talk, but after my name was called, I had to cut the conversation short.

I was ready to see the doctor. My weight was 184 pounds due to the Prednisone pills I was taking. My blood pressure was up somewhat that morning due to the swelling I was having.

Gout

When I saw the doctor, and showed him my finger, he was very concerned. He said he wanted to find out if the swelling in my finger was lupus related or gout related. He said, "If the fluid from your finger comes out thick, it is definitely gout." He explained that the procedure would be done right there in the office. I asked the doctor, "When will I get the results back?" His response to me was, "Right now." I was excited to hear how fast I would get the results back, so I immediately consented to have it done.

How Was the Procedure Done?

The doctor deadened my finger where the swelling was. He then inserted the needle into my left ring finger for just a second and the syringe pulled out some fluid that looked thick from the swollen area. Then, the fluid was put into the tube. A sample piece of glass was also smeared with the fluid to be checked.

The doctor immediately came right back and told me that it was not lupus related. He told me that I had gout. I was so shocked that I had to ask the doctor, "How in the world did I get gout?" He said, "You probably have too much uric acid in your body that is not coming out like it should." He told me to wait about six more weeks until my next appointment, so that a new medication could be given to get rid of some of the uric acid in my body.

When I came back out into the waiting room area, where my children were, I explained to them everything that had happened. I had to wait for my prescriptions to be written up and then filled when I got home. I also had to get some blood work done at the lab that day, as well as give some urine. As I continued speaking with a few of the ladies that were still there at the Lupus Clinic, I told them that I was writing a book about lupus. They were all very excited to hear that and said they could not wait to read my book. I explained to them that my oldest daughter was the one who encouraged me to write my lupus story and the challenges I had to face. I told them that I have been writing my lupus story daily since I was a very young girl. And now that I was sixty years old and living with lupus, it was time for my story to be told. I told them that my life was not all pretty, but it is my own true story. We all exchanged telephone numbers and said we would keep in touch.

Reflections: How I felt that day of my Clinic Appointment

As I awoke that morning on September 11, 2012 before going to the Lupus Clinic, I put some very positive energy out there. I had already felt that, no matter what, it was going to be a beautiful day and indeed it was. Everyone that I came in contact with was very nice, friendly, warm, and courteous. I felt so well taken care of by the doctors at Grady Hospital, and I met some very nice people from the lupus support group. They were all looking forward to reading my story. What more could I have asked for?

Renal Clinic Appointment - 10/3/12

On the morning of October 3, 2012, I was on my way to Grady Hospital to see the renal doctors regarding my kidneys.

It was a very nice Wednesday morning, and I had just arrived at Grady Hospital. My clinic appointment was at 11:00 AM. Again, it was not crowded at all, so I knew that I would be seen very quickly. The two doctors that were in the room with me checked my lab work and said that things were looking good.

I was currently taking two 5 mg tablets of Prednisone daily, one 25 mg tablet of Hydrochlorothiazide, and one 40 mg tablet of Lisinopril—only when my blood pressure was extremely high. I was explaining to the doctors that on September 22, 2012, I stopped taking my Mychophe-nolate (Cellcept) medication because I did not like the way I was feeling. I told them that it made me feel really off-balanced when I was walking. I had been on that medication since 2010. The doctors said that since things were looking good and I was feeling much better, it was okay. Plus, they saw that I had been on that medication for a good while.

I was not taking my Lisinopril 40 mg tablet everyday, but only as needed when my blood pressure became elevated. I was still taking the 25 mg tablet of Hydrochlorothiazide daily, as well as my two 5 mg tablets of Prednisone daily. The renal doctors explained that I should definitely stop taking the Hydrochlorothiazide 25 mg tablet. They told me to start taking one 40 mg tablet of Lisinopril everyday. I was surprised when they said that because I had never done that before.

The doctors were looking over my hospital records and saw that my last flare-up was with gout when I was seen at the Rheumatology Clinic.

An Allergic Reaction

Well, after my appointment with the Renal Clinic, I was now on one 40 mg tablet of Lisinopril and one 10 mg tablet of Prednisone.

After taking Lisinopril everyday as instructed, it was not agreeing with me at all. I had an allergic reaction to that medication. My right leg was paining me so severely that the bones in my body were aching. The pain was so bad that it kept me up all hours of the night and I was not even able to get a good night's sleep. I was also experiencing very severe lower back pain, severe pelvic pain, lower abdominal pain, hip pain, and joint pain. I was no good. I was in so much traumatic pain everyday that I could not believe this was happening to me—especially not all at the same time. Therefore, I started to immediately do some research and found out that other people have also experienced some of the same things that I was experiencing.

So, on Monday, October 8, 2012, I stopped taking the Lisinopril medication altogether. I called the Rheumatology Clinic every Tuesday and was constantly leaving messages for someone to get back to me, but no one ever called me back. I was not well and suffering with so much pain throughout my entire body.

On October 30, 2012, when I had a lupus appointment to see the doctor, I was in constant pain and suffering and was just trying to make it to the hospital. So, in the wee hours of the morning, I started calling some taxicabs, but there were none available that early. I was in so much pain and trying to figure out what I was going to do next. Christopher had to leave for school by 6:00 AM, in order to make it to his first class and my doctors appointment was at 10:30 AM.

I told Christopher and Christel that I had no choice but to drive. It was very, very dark outside, which was good. I was feeling too sick; I could barely even walk. Before getting into the car, Christel put a pillow on the seat of the car and another pillow for my lower back. This crisis was one of the hardest I had to endure while driving. To top it all off, I could only drive using just my left hand because everything on the right side of my body was in turmoil. Seeing how much pain that I was in, my son looked at me and started crying as he sat in the front seat of the car next to me. He tried rubbing my legs, but the pain was unbearable and it was not letting up. I prayed aloud that we all made it safely to the train station and we did. I was able to find a parking space because it was still very early.

The next task for me was getting out of the car and trying to make it up the street. I could barely walk, but I made it. I was so glad that it was still dark outside and not too many people were on the street to see the condition that I was in. When we got in the train, I sat down by the window and started rubbing my legs. After Christopher got off the train to his destination, Christel and I proceeded on. When our stop came we got off and had to take another train, just one stop before reaching our final destination.

We arrived at Grady Hospital at 6:30 AM. I was in so much pain in the elevator as my daughter and I headed up to the 12th floor of the Lupus Clinic. Even though my appointment was at 10:30 AM, I was glad that I was early. All I wanted to do was sit down! I informed the front desk receptionist that I had been calling and calling the hospital for weeks and leaving messages, but no one ever called me back. The receptionist was shocked because she said she put the messages on the doctor's desk. She saw that I was completely bent over and could barely walk, so she immediately clocked me in at 7:00 AM. I appreciated that very much. She told me that she would also make sure that whichever doctor came in first, would see me.

As I was being seen, I explained to the doctors that I had been suffering for far too long—since I was last seen on October 3, 2012, at the Renal Clinic. I was telling them that I had been leaving message after message and that no one called me back. The doctors who were attending to me were so surprised to hear that no one responded to any of my telephone calls. They apologized to me for what I was going through. I was telling them that all of this happened to me when the renal doctors decided to put me on a 40 mg dose of Lisinopril that I had to take every day. I also told them that when I started doing some research, I found out that there were other people who have experienced some of the same symptoms as I did on that dose.

When I was on the table being examined by the doctors, they wanted me to show them the areas of my body that were painful. I explained that my pelvic bones were aching and my back felt like it was splitting in half. I told them that my legs, from the knees on down, felt numb, and that every joint throughout the right side of my body had been attacked by the pain. I explained that I was suffering with very severe pain, but nothing was wrong with the left side of my body.

Lumbosacral Radiculopathy

After all of the symptoms were reviewed by the doctor, they told me that I had lumbosacral radiculopathy. I asked what that meant and the doctor said, that

I have a pinched nerve, or nerves, in the lower back (lumbosacral area). She said when that happens, I may experience weakness in my legs and not be able to stand up on my toes. She also said that what I was going through was not going to be an easy fix and would take some time because all of that did not happen to me overnight.

At that same time, I was also experiencing severe gout pain. I asked the doctors, "Where in the world did I get this gout from anyway?" The doctors told me that my gout probably came from the different medications I was taking. I asked them to please give me something for the gout. The doctor told me that being on too many medications was not good at all and that if I started on another new medication, I would probably die. She said that first, she wanted to get a hold of what was causing all of the pain that I was experiencing. I understood clearly what the doctor was saying.

I was then given a prescription for a 300 mg capsule of Gabapentin to be taken by mouth three times a day to help relieve the lower back pain. I was still taking my one 10 mg tablet of Prednisone to help calm the gout down; and for my high blood pressure, I was told to fill the prescription for a 50 mg tablet of Losartan Potassium, but to not take it just yet.

After my clinic visit was over, it was still very early. The doctor decided that I should have some lab work done, as well as have some x-rays taken of my bones and spine. On my next lupus visit, I would get the results of everything.

I had my blood drawn first. Then, I had the x-rays done. The technician told me how sorry he was when he had to pull my legs in so many different directions in order for him to have accurate pictures taken. He took so many pictures that I could not even keep up with it anymore. I cried and muddled through that horrible ordeal. I was so mad because I had no idea just how painful that was going to be for me. If I would have known ahead of time that I was going to be in that much pain, I probably would have waited until the pain medication was already in my system.

It was finally time for me to leave the hospital. That was such a long morning for me, and I had no idea how I was going to make it through. Since my car was already parked at the station, I was able to wait for Christopher to meet up with Christel and I. It was good because Christopher had left school at the same time we left the hospital. Once I was in the car, I was still experiencing so much pain. Christel said to me, "Mommy, despite all of that pain you were going through, you really did good today." I looked at my daughter and said, "Christel, by the grace of God was how I made it." We waited in front of the train station for no more than fifteen minutes before Christopher arrived. The first thing that Christopher asked when he got in the car was, "Mommy, what did the doctors say today?" I told him that I had lumbosacral radiculopathy. I explained that it meant that I had a pinched nerve. I also told him that the doctor prescribed a nerve medication for me to take three times a day, called Gabapentin. He said, "Oh Wow, I wonder how that happened." I said, "Christopher, I have no idea." My son told me that I did very well after everything I had been through. I told him the same thing I had said to Christel…that it was only by the grace of God that I was able to make it to the hospital. I also told my children that it was a good thing I did not know ahead of time the pain that I would have to go through having those x-rays taken because that was something I would not want to repeat.

While I was still in severe agony and pain, I made it to the pharmacy near my home. They saw the excruciating pain that I was in, so they did not let me wait at all. My prescriptions were filled immediately. I thanked them so much for doing that for me.

My next appointment to see the doctor would not be until the New Year of January 2013.

After I was seen at the Lupus Clinic, I could not believe that, by the evening of that same day, I was feeling even worse than ever. I was experiencing even more pain than before. I kept asking myself, *How can someone's body endure so much suffering and excruciating pain like this?* None of the medications were helping. Being on that 10 mg tablet of Prednisone for the gout did not do anything, and my body was feeling worse than ever. I was unable to breathe properly and knew that something had to be done immediately.

In Emergency at Grady Memorial Hospital

That very next day, on October 31, 2012, my daughter, Christine, decided to rush me to Grady Memorial Hospital since I had just taken blood tests and x-rays at the hospital the day before.

After arriving at the hospital, they took me immediately because they saw that I could not breathe and was bent over in so much pain. The pregnant woman at the desk asked me what was going on. I told the woman that when I started taking Lisinopril on October 3rd, I did not like the way it made me feel. Then, on October 8th, I felt so horrible, that I had to stop taking it altogether. I also told her that this was the after effects of what I was going through. The nice woman said that she heard a lot of people talking about Lisinopril and what they were going through as well. She just shook her head. She told my son, who was also with my oldest daughter and I, that he could come with us while I was being escorted to one of the rooms for immediate attention. The young lady did not want me to wait at all. I appreciated the fast response she gave and the kindness she showed.

When I saw the doctors in the emergency room, I told them that I had just been seen at the Lupus Clinic yesterday and they took complete blood work and also x-rays of my spine. The doctors were glad to hear that my x-rays were already done and that they did not have to do that. They quickly got a hold of my x-rays. The doctor who was looking at my x-rays told me that he also went through the same exact thing that I was going through. He said, "You have a pinched nerve." He told me the exact same thing that the doctors at the Lupus Clinic said to me: that this was not going to be an easy fix.

He asked me for the medications I was taking from the Lupus Clinic. I told him that the day before, I was instructed by the doctor to start taking a Gabapentin 300 mg capsule by mouth three times a day. The doctor in the emergency room told me that since Gabapentin takes about two weeks before it really takes effect in the body, he had to prescribe Ibuprofen—an 800 mg tablet—to be taken every eight hours for the pain I was having. He told me that was all he could do at the time because there was going to be a waiting period.

Doctor Made a Phone Call to My Home – 11/3/12

After my visit with the lupus doctors back on October 30, 2012—and after I let them know that none of the doctors called me back when I was sick—it was very nice to see that one of the doctors took it upon herself to call me at home on Saturday, November 3, 2012. She told me that she was thinking about me and wanted to give me an update on the tests that I had taken.

She told me that she saw a little something in the x-rays that I took. I immediately told her that, when I returned home after being seen at the clinic on October 30th, I was feeling so bad that my daughter had to rush me to the emergency room at Grady that very next day. I told her that the doctor in emergency gave me a prescription for Ibuprofen at 800 mg to be taken as needed for pain. She quickly said, "Please do not take any Ibuprofen tablets that the emergency room has prescribed for you." She told me that it was not good for me and that I should not take it. I was really surprised to hear her say that. She explained to me step-by-step the medications that I should continue to take. They were: Gabapentin 300 mg capsules three times a day, Oxycodone 10 mg/Acetamino-phen 325 mg tablet every eight hours as needed for pain, the generic for Percocet 10/325 mg, and there would be no refills remaining for that prescription. I thanked the doctor very much for calling me and continued to take the medications that we talked about.

Gout Continued to Get Worse 11/5/12

It was November 5, 2012, the month that I would never forget. I experienced the worse gout flare-up that one could ever imagine. When the gout attacked my feet, that was one of the worst types of pain ever. My toes became red and inflamed, and it was so unbearable that I could not even walk.

Then, on November 8, 2012, I noticed that my left leg was stinging and felt so tight and numb. Also, on November 9, 2012, both legs were becoming so tight that I was really getting scared. None of the prescribed medications were working for me. My whole body was in so much turmoil that I could no longer use my right hand at all. The entire right side of my body was just not working for me. I was suffering in the worse way possible. I dreaded going to bed at night because it was so hard for me to sleep. I would use at least four pillows to try and get some relief, but I still felt worse than ever. Nothing was working for me at all. I would just moan and groan every night until the morning came. I did not have a decent night's sleep for about a month and a half. During the week of November 12th, my legs were no longer working for me. When I had to use the bathroom, I found it difficult to walk from my bedroom to the bathroom without falling or needing to hold on to something.

Trying to Prepare for the Thanksgiving Holiday

It was the week of Thanksgiving and, believe it or not, with all that I was going through, I was trying my best to prepare for the holiday. It was going to be a very intimate day with my sister, her son, and my family. The bad thing was, I could no longer use my right hand. My hand swelled up so bad that it looked like a plastic glove filled up with water. No matter what, I still tried my best to cook and do whatever I had to do. With the help of my children, I knew that everything would be fine.

The day came. It was November 22, 2012, the morning of Thanksgiving. I was feeling horrible. My hand had really swollen up bad and I had no more energy left to give. I could barely walk. I just wanted to lie down on the bed that was in my living room and even that felt hard for me to do.

When everyone arrived, they saw how weak I looked. They even saw, for the very first time, that my hand was very badly swollen and I could hardly move my body. My sister, Claudette, and my daughter, Christine, told me that if I wanted to go to the hospital, which I was not looking forward to at that very moment, they were more than willing to go with me. I told them that since it was Thanksgiving Day, and I was so out of it, I did not feel like going anywhere. I told them that, if I do not feel any better the next day, then I would definitely go. Just having my family with me was good enough for me.

It was the day after Thanksgiving on November 23, 2012. When I woke up that morning and tried to lift my head off of the pillow to get up, I could not do it. My body was shutting down on me, and I was unable to stand up or walk at all. My children have never witnessed me in that condition. When Christel woke up and walked into my room, she could not hold back her tears. Christopher tried to console her, and I just looked at both of them as I was lying on the bed.

At that moment, I had to use the bathroom, so Christopher got a bucket for me to use. When he tried to help me up from the bed, I fell. I had no strength to even help myself. My body was feeling like dead weight, with nothing but pain—I could not bear it.

Christopher and I did not know what to do because Christel had already left for work. Christopher cried out to me, shaking his head, "Mommy, I cannot do this anymore!" I told him to call Christine.

Christine went to get my sister. When they arrived, they came upstairs to the bedroom where I was still laying. They saw the physical state I was in. They alerted me that an ambulance must be called. I could not say anything to them. I was suffering and in too much pain. Since my entire body was completely shutting down on me, the slightest touch to my body was excruciating.

The Ambulance Arrived

When the ambulance and the fire department arrived, there were at least four to five very nice people that came into my bedroom to assist me. They saw that I was in very bad shape when they tried to move me out of my bed. I was yelling out to them, asking that they please do not drop me. They told me that they were going to put a sheet underneath my body to lift me off of the bed and into the wheelchair. I continued to moan and groan as I yelled out to them, "Please do not drop me." I really felt that if they would have dropped me, I would not be any good anymore—like my body would have just crumbled.

When the paramedics finally lifted me off of the bed and into the wheelchair, I told them to please make sure that the wheelchair did not hit the steps when we went down the stairs. I told them to please lift the wheelchair up because the slightest touch to any part of my body would be too painful for me to bear. I was glad that they were able to accomplish that. When they had to get me off of the chair and onto the stretcher, I was still moaning and groaning until I got into the ambulance. After that, the paramedics called Piedmont Hospital and alerted them that we were on our way. Claudette was sitting up front with the driver, I was lying down in the back, and my daughter, Christine, was driving behind us.

Arriving at Piedmont Hospital

When we arrived at Piedmont Hospital, they were already waiting for us and saw the terrible shape that I was in. They wasted no time and immediately started working on me. At that time, I was delirious. I had chills and a fever of about 104.4. My body was in so much turmoil that the doctor put IVs in both of my arms. They took about ten tubes of blood from my right arm and had a very hard time getting blood from my left arm. When they finally found a vein, my blood came out so profusely that it was dripping on the hospital floor. I was lying in the bed, so cold that I had started trembling and my teeth were chattering uncontrollably. I asked for more blankets. The doctors told me that I could not have any covers because they wanted my fever to break. I was so mad! After the doctor and his team saw that things were moving in the right direction, I was told that I would be okay and was admitted for further treatment.

I was put into a very nice private room where the nurses carefully monitored me around-the-clock. They were constantly checking my blood pressure because it was very high. When they began administering pain medications intravenously, that was the biggest relief for me.

My sister, Claudette, was surprised that she was not even tired after staying up for at least twenty-seven hours because she was the type of person that always needed to get her rest. I told her, "When your heart is in the right place, God can give you strength that you never knew was possible." When Claudette and Christine saw that I looked very sleepy, relaxed, and comfortable, they decided that they would go home and get some rest. My diagnosis was a very high fever, hypertension, gout, a pinched nerve, acute renal failure, and Lupus (SLE). This was the worst diagnosis that I had ever received from a doctor all at the same time.

I was receiving so many medications around-the-clock to get my body back in shape. They were: Norvasc 5 mg (given to me that Sunday morning at 11:30 AM. After taking it, my blood pressure was still very high and did not go down.); Gabapentin 300 mg (which was a capsule that I took three times a day. That medication was for my pinched nerve.); Hydralazine 10 mg (started at 5:00 AM. That medication was given to me intravenously every six hours.); Lovenox 40 mg (which was a blood thinner. After being in the hospital before, I did not like the feeling of needles being put in my thighs and buttocks every single day. So, I refused to take it.); Colchicine 0.6 mg (for gout, the doctor did not want it administered to me intravenously; therefore, I received a tiny lavendar pill—the size of rice, but fatter) that was taken by mouth twice a day.); Pepcid 20 mg tablet (that was taken by mouth twice a day with my meals. That tablet was to coat my stomach from all of the medications I had been taking.); Cyclobenzaprine 5 mg tablet (to help with my continuous muscle spasms. It really helped me. I took it three times a day, but only as needed.); Oxycodone HCL 5 mg tablet (taken by mouth every six hours. It was taken as needed for pain.); Vancomycin (given every eighteen hours intravenously to treat bacterial infections.); and finally, Zosyn (given every eight hours to treat a wide variety of bacterial infections.)

After all of those medications were given to me, I was able to have something that I had not had in a very long time…and that was a good night's sleep.

As I awoke on the morning of November 24, 2012, I was looking over the hospital's menu and requested that I be put on the low sodium diet. The nurse provided me with the cafeteria's extension number to call and make my request. After going over the menu with me, within one hour, my breakfast was delivered to my room. The food was excellent! I really appreciated the way they calculated the sodium intake of the food that I received throughout the course of the day.

Even though I had been through a very rough time, and all of the medications that I was on, I was so glad to be alive. I learned from the doctor that when I experience gout flares, I should not take any water pills of any kind because it would only make the gout worse. That was why, when I was admitted into the hospital, they immediately took me off the Bumetanide tablet and the Hydrochlorothiazide tablet that I was taking once daily.

I was given a medication list to follow once I was discharged on November 28, 2012. It was a new day and a new beginning for me. The at-home medications that I continued were: a 300 mg Gabapentin Capsule that I took three times a day and my 10 mg Prednisone pill that I took once a day. The new medications I started when I got home were: Amlodipine Besylate, which was a 10 mg tablet that was taken once a day; Colchicine, a 0.6 mg tablet that was taken two times a day; Cyclobenzaprine, which was a 10 mg tablet that was taken three times a day; Famotidine, a 20 mg tablet that was taken two times a day with my meals; and Hydralazine, a 25 mg tablet that was taken every eight hours.

I did not take Hydralazine when my systolic blood pressure (the top number) was less than 110. I took Oxycodone, which was a 5 mg tablet taken every six hours.

I was instructed to stop taking the Acetaminophen/Oxycodone tablet that I took every eight hours as needed for pain. That tablet included 325 mgs of Acetaminopen and 10 mgs of Oxycodone. I did, however, stop taking all water pills.

On December 6, 2012, at exactly 5:32 PM, I was right back at the Piedmont Hospital emergency room because I was experiencing very bad joint pains. After seeing the doctor, I was given a higher dose of Prednisone at 40 mgs that I needed to fill when I got home. The doctor instructed me to taper off the Prednisone every two weeks until I was down to only 10 mgs.

That very next day on December 7, 2012, I received a telephone call from Piedmont Hospital. They were glad to hear that I was doing okay and feeling much better.

Christel's Accomplishment

Christel's Cosmetology teacher, Mrs. Harris—that she'd had since high school—was an excellent teacher. Even after Christel graduated, Mrs. Harris extended herself out to my daughter so that she could get the extra help she needed as she prepared for the cosmetology test.

The day after Christmas, on December 26, 2012, Christel was scheduled to take the Georgia State Board of Cosmetology's practical exam. She was so nervous! That test was all hands-on. Christine, Christopher, and I were there to support Christel as we waited for her to finish the exam. After a few hours had passed, Christel came down off the elevator from where we were seated and showed us her paper. We were so excited when we saw that she had passed! Christel said that she felt so stressed out. All she wanted to do was go home and lie down. She now held the title of Master Cosmetologist. That license would enable her to work in not just one field of Cosmetology, but in all of the different areas. That was such a wonderful gift and a way to end 2012!

After the holidays were over and we were in the New Year of 2013, my daughter could not wait to contact Mrs. Harris. She called Mrs. Harris during school hours and told her the good news. Mrs. Harris was so happy and excited for Christel. Mrs. Harris told Christel how proud she was of her and immediately shared the good news with the other students while Christel was on the telephone.

Lupus Clinic Appointments - Grady Memorial Hospital

On May 14, 2013, Christel and I were on our way to the Lupus Clinic at Grady Memorial Hospital. When we arrived, I could already see that it was going to be a very long day. There were not too many doctors there that morning. After sitting there for at least two and a half to three hours, my name was finally called. When I sat down with the doctors, they looked over my chart records. Their concern was that my blood pressure was very high. They decided that they did not want to change the blood pressure medications that I was on. I was told to keep a record of my blood pressure daily until my next clinic visit in the beginning of July.

Christopher and I were on our way to the Lupus Clinic at Grady Memorial Hospital on the morning of July 2, 2013. When we arrived, I was glad that we would not have to wait too long to see the doctor. As my name was called, Christopher decided that he wanted to come in the room with me to hear what the doctors had to say. At that time, there were two lady doctors in the room looking over my chart records. The biggest problem that I had was that my blood pressure was still very high. Then, I explained to the doctors that my gout had been flaring up from time to time. I told them that I had eliminated all foods that contained high fructose corn syrup from my diet. After doing that, I saw that it really helped. The doctor advised me to take three medications for my gout. They were Allopurinol, a 100 mg tablet to be taken once a day; Colcrys, a 0.6 mg tablet to be taken once a day; and a 10 mg Prednisone pill to be taken once a day for pain.

For my blood pressure, I had to take: Amlodipine Besylate, a 10 mg tablet to be taken once a day; Losartan Potassium, a 50 mg tablet to be taken once a day; and Metoprolol Tartrate, a 50 mg tablet to be taken once a day.

I was scheduled to see the doctor at the Lupus Clinic on September 3, 2013, but due to my son's college commitments, I was unable to come and had to reschedule.

Portfolio Show and Awards Ceremony

On Thursday, September 12, 2013, it was Christopher's last day of school at The Art Institute of Atlanta, as well as his Portfolio Show and Awards Ceremony. We had to be there from 11:00 AM all the way until 8:00 PM. When we arrived, there was a Portfolio Show set-up. Then, we had to break for lunch.

Immediately following, there was a Portfolio Show Preview and Awards Ceremony. My son could not believe that the portfolio he worked so hard on won "Best in Show" for Illustration and Design. The Art Institute of Atlanta presented Christopher with the Best Portfolio Award for Illustration, Bachelor of Fine Arts. I was so proud of what my son had accomplished.

After that, we went back to my son's designated room where his Portfolio, along with his award, was displayed. We saw so many beautiful portfolios displayed by the students. Later that evening, they had a private meeting that was held for the students only—where they met and talked with some top professionals in their field. After that long, long day, my son said his good-byes to everyone.

When we got home, we started talking about everything. Christopher learned so much during those years in school and owes it to the teachers who believed in him. He was especially grateful for having a teacher like Mrs. Bolling. Christopher was in Mrs. Bolling's Graphic Design and Portfolio class. Mrs. Bolling saw that Christopher was talented, had a strong content of character, and worked hard to make things happen. Christopher was forever grateful to Mrs. Bolling for believing in him and not letting him go unnoticed. We also talked about those long hours at night doing schoolwork. It paid off for him. His goal was to graduate with a straight 100% in all of his classes and he did exactly that.

My Godmother Passed Away

My Godmother, Mrs. Salome Finney, was very sick and her health had taken a toll on her. On November 25, 2013, she passed away at the age of 92. Her service took place on Sunday, December 1, 2013 in the Bronx, New York. I will always remember those beautiful memories we shared; especially during 1999 when she came down to Atlanta with my mother and her older sister to visit with my children and I. She gave me a small square pillow that read: All Things Grow With Love.

Lupus Clinic Appointment – 12/3/13

On December 3, 2013, Christel went with me to Grady Memorial Hospital. I had eaten a lot of food during that Thanksgiving holiday, so I knew my weight was going to go up. When we arrived, I immediately got my lab work done first and then headed back to the Lupus Clinic. At that time, the clinic was full. I could not wait to hear what the doctor was going to say to me that day. After my name was called, Christel and I proceeded back to the doctor's office. I sat down with the doctor and explained my concerns. I told him that, due to the amount of lab work I have been taking—as well as all of my medications—it had been very hard on me to come to the clinic often. I told him that all of my medical expenses have been out-of-pocket. He understood my concerns.

After he looked over my records and saw the results of the lab tests I had taken earlier that morning, he was pleased with the results. He had another doctor come into the office to see me, as well. That doctor spoke with me, examined me, and discussed my Lupus Nephritis and gout. She gave me a prescription for a higher dose of Allopurinol (Zyloprim), which was a 300 mg tablet to be taken by mouth once a day. I continued taking Colchicine (Colcrys), a 0.6 mg tablet that I took only as needed. Those medications were for the gout. Then, for my high blood pressure, I took Amlodipine (Norvasc), a 10 mg tablet to be taken by mouth once a day. Then, the Losartan (Cozaar) was increased to a 100 mg tablet to be taken by mouth daily. My Prednisone (Deltasone) was decreased by taking a 5 mg tablet and breaking it in half, to be taken by mouth daily. We also discussed the vitamins that I was already taking and the doctor said it was okay. I had a very good doctor's visit.

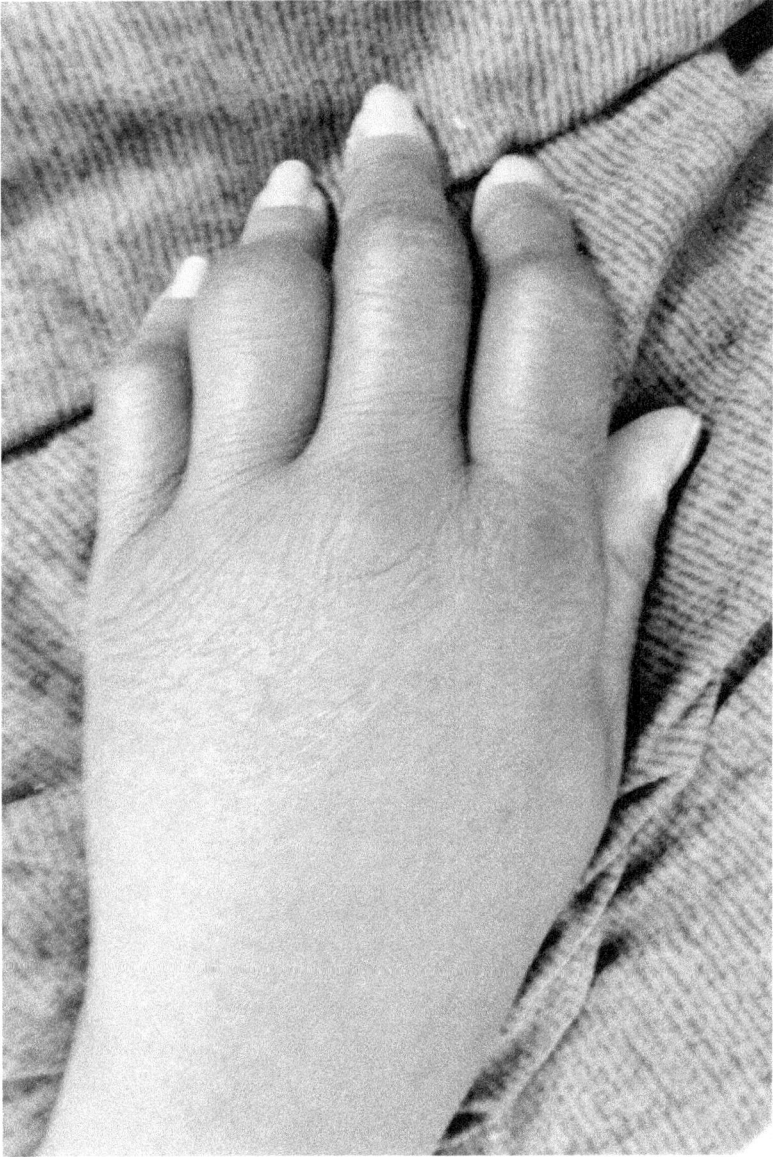

Lupus Flare-up: My hand was so badly swollen.

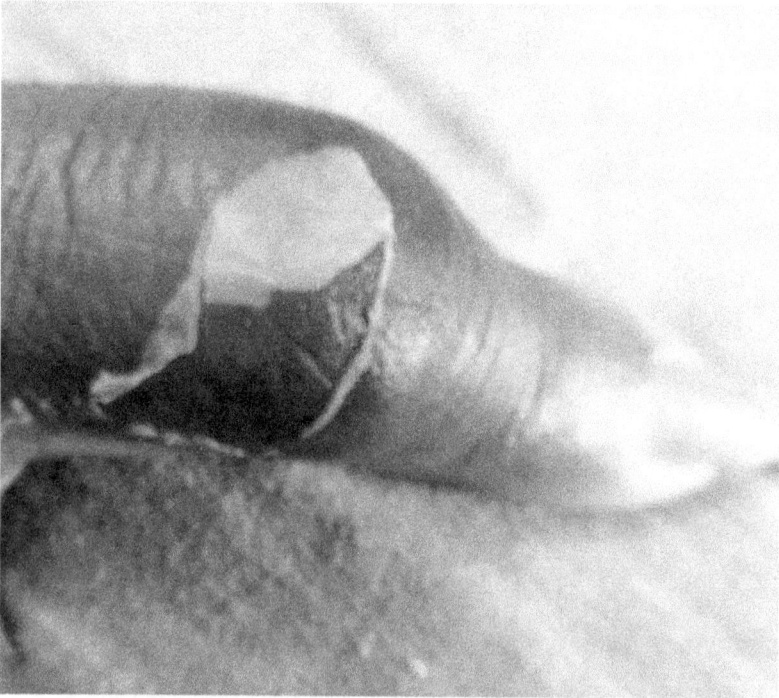

My finger was badly swollen and started to peel.

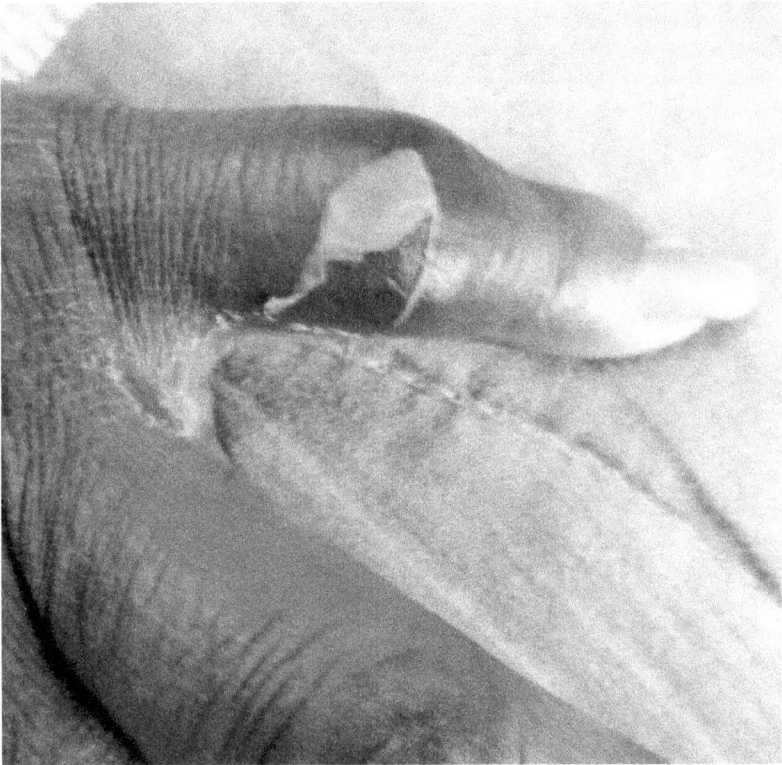

The swelling was gradually going down.

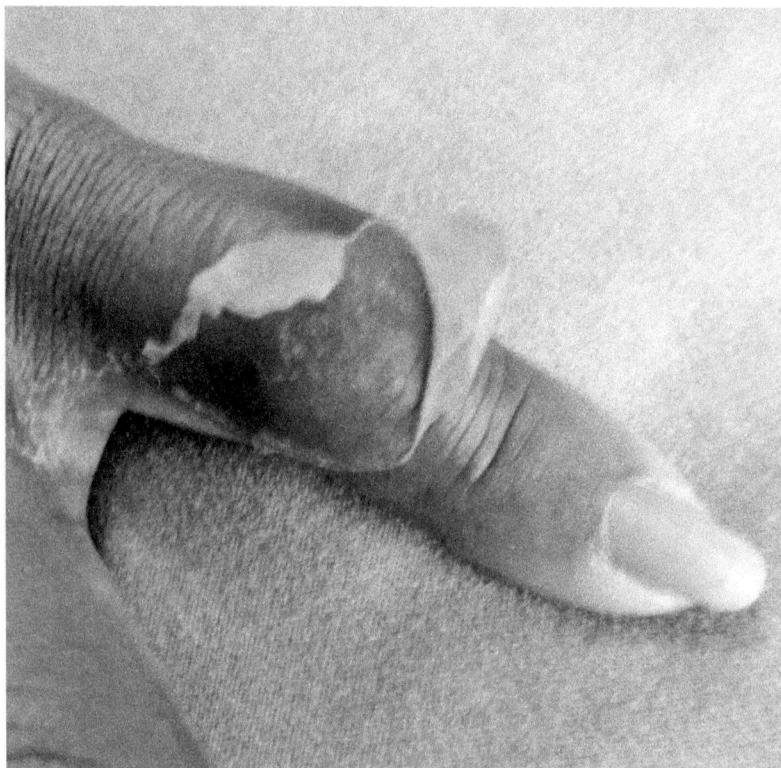

My skin continued to peel.

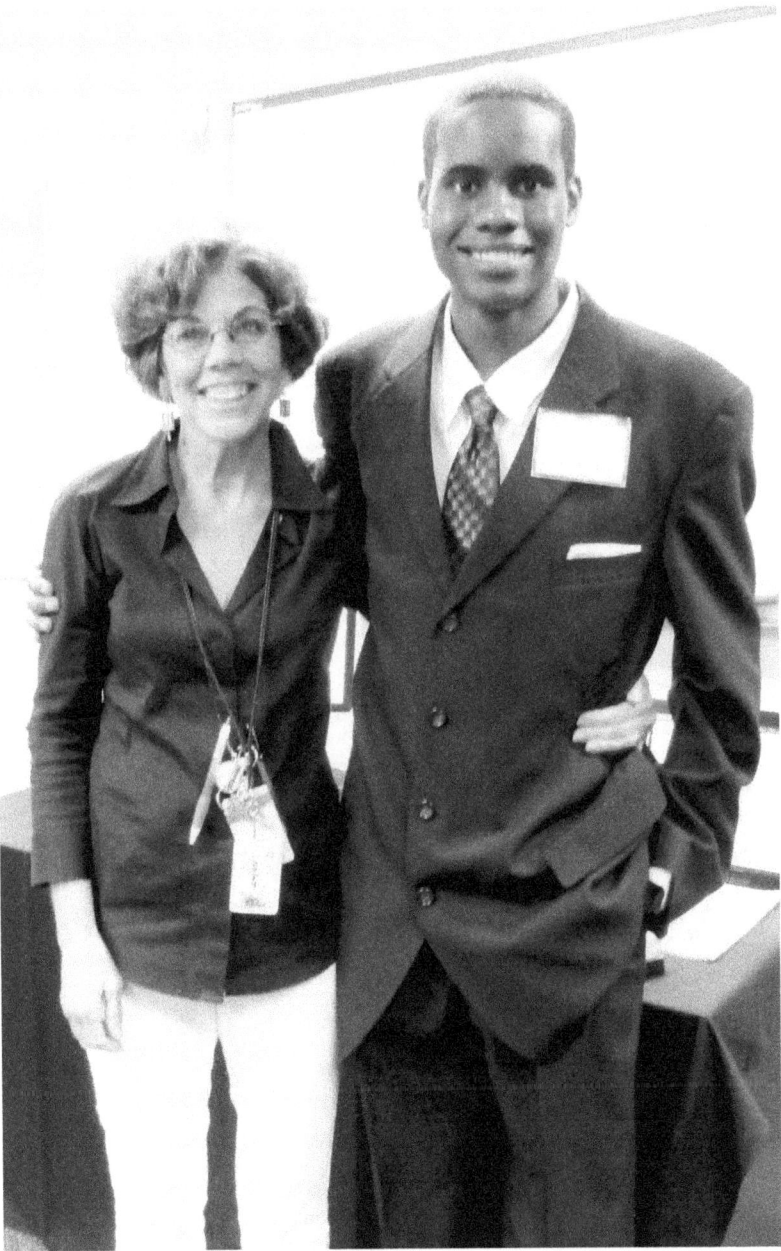

Portfolio Show and Awards Ceremony - September 12, 2013
My son, Christopher, and his teacher, Mrs. Bolling.

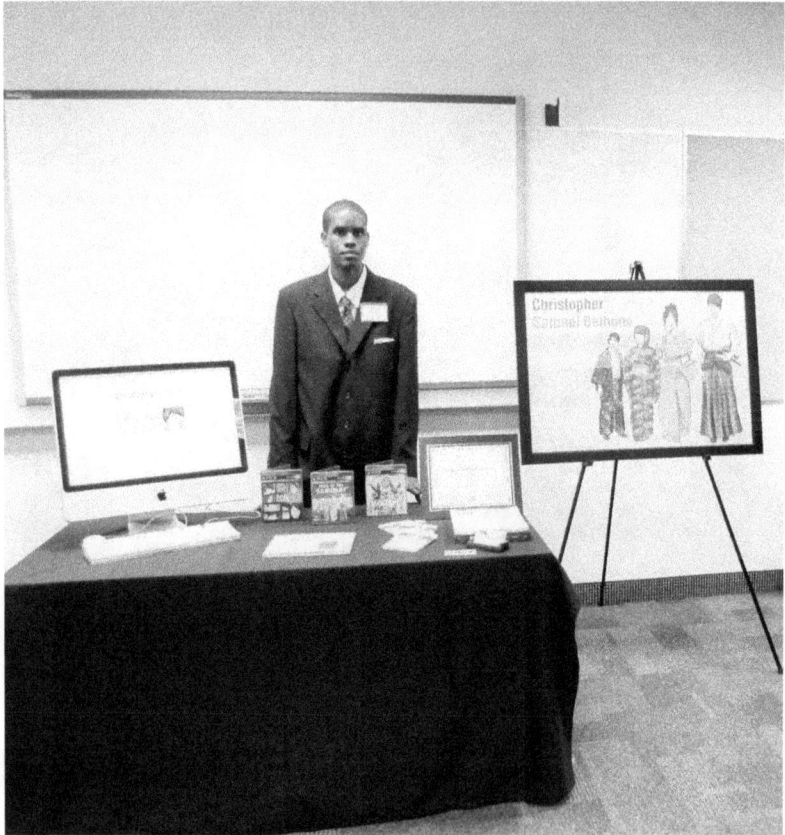

My son, Christopher won "Best in Show"- September 12, 2013
He was looking on as everyone started entering the room.

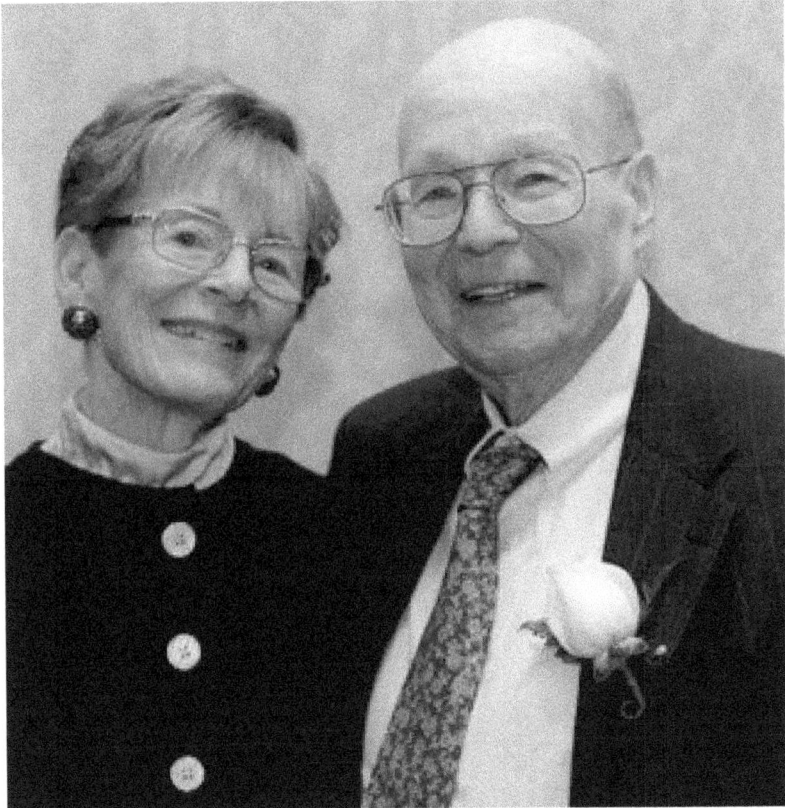

Dr. Christine Lawrence at a 2013 Gala Awards Dinner for her husband, Dr. Milford Fulop. Both received an award for their combined service of 100 years at Jacobi Hospital, Bronx New York.

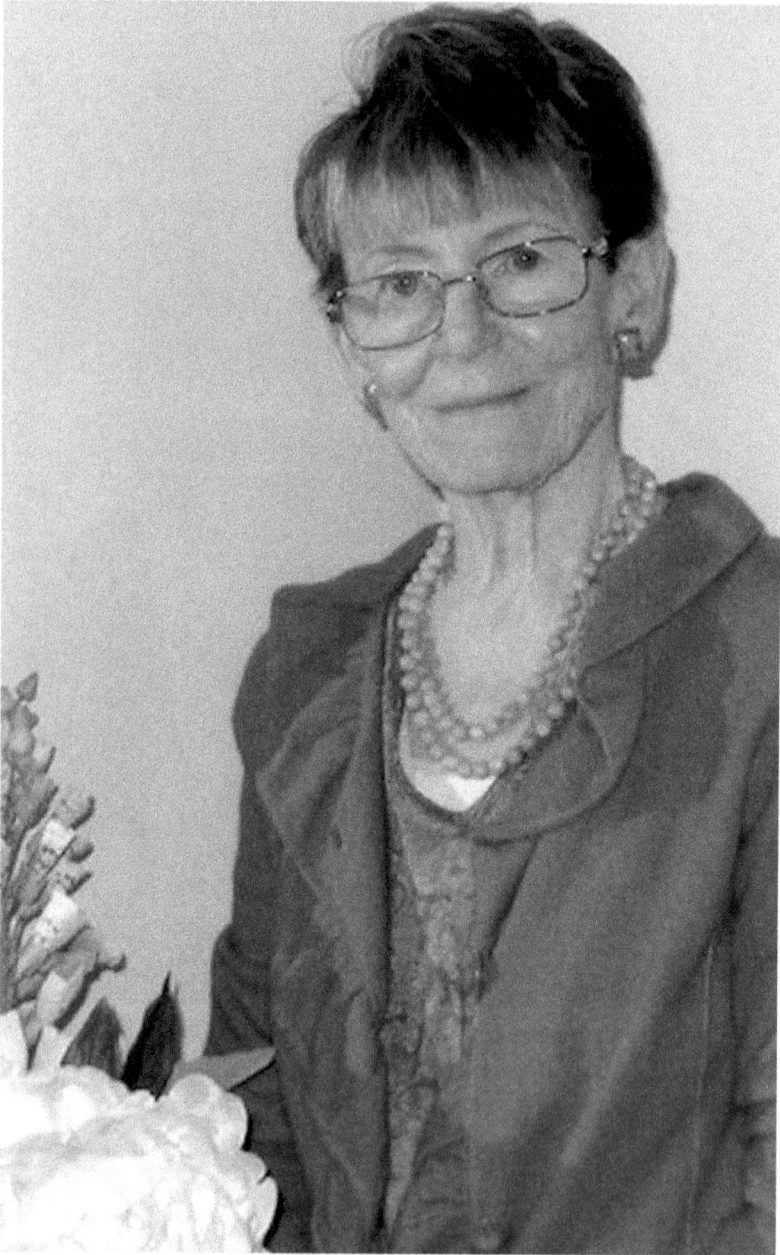

This is a current picture of Dr. Christine Lawrence.

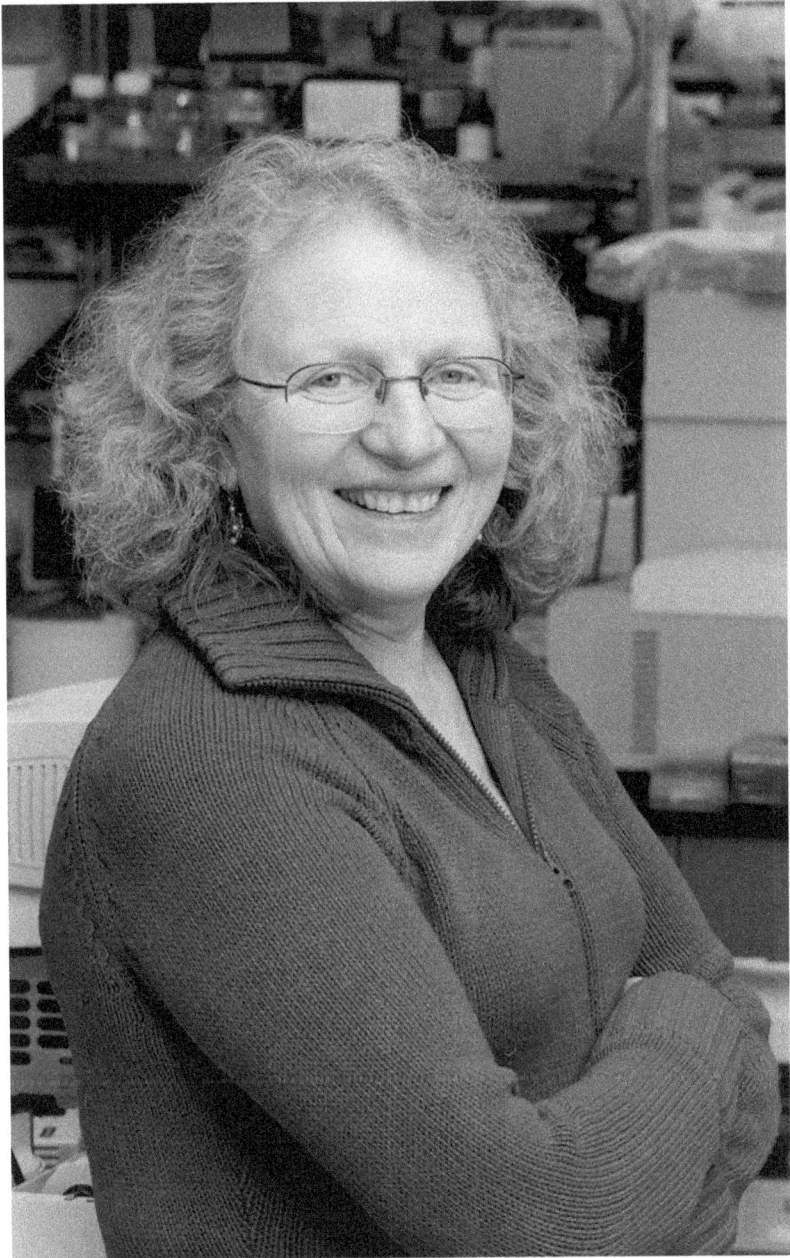

This is a current picture of Dr. Betty Diamond.

CHAPTER 10

A WEDDING TO REMEMBER

On Christmas Eve, we wanted to keep the tradition going by spending quality time with family at my home. Plus, I always enjoy cooking for everyone. We usually "chill out," have good conversation, and eat all night long.

Well, this particular Christmas Eve was special. My daughter, Christine, and her boyfriend, Garland, were sitting down at the dining room table. I was surprised to hear the news. My daughter announced that she and Garland were looking forward to getting married on October 18, 2014. We were all very happy to hear that great news! The first thing that I asked was, "Who picked that specific date?" They said that it just felt right and it did not conflict with their busy schedules. They both agreed, that date was the perfect time for their wedding.

I told Christine that, even though she did not realize it, this particular date was the same day as Dr.

Lawrence's birthday. She said, "Really!" She could not believe it. I told her that Dr. Lawrence was going to be so surprised that she picked October 18th as their wedding day. I knew in my heart, that was the perfect date. I thought to myself, *Look at how life comes around full circle.* My life as a young person changed when I met Dr. Lawrence; I named Christine after Dr. Lawrence; and Christine and Garland were getting married on Dr. Lawrence's birthday. The amazing thing about it all was that they said the date just felt right to them. That was so wonderful to hear, and it was a good way to end the year.

Entering a New Year

As we entered the New Year of 2014, I wished for a year of change. Too Many people were sick and dying each and everyday due to a lack of health insurance. Medicaid still needed to be expanded to those that really need it. I was so grateful that the doctor listened to what I was saying at my last clinic appointment in December, concerning my lack of medical insurance.

Lupus Clinic Appointment – 6/3/14

On June 3, 2014, Christopher came with me when I was seen during my visit at the Lupus Clinic. My blood pressure was a little high that morning and my medications had not quite kicked in for that early morning appointment. On that visit, the doctor had me take x-rays on both of my hands, to see just how much the gout had affected me. I was not experiencing any joint pain at that time, and I was told to continue taking the same medications from when I was last seen in December 2013. I was not looking forward to any more gout flares any time soon.

Christine and Garland's Wedding Was Approaching

Christine and Garland's wedding was slowly approaching. Garland's sister, Andrea, was the event planner. That helped make things so much easier for Christine and Garland, and also made it so much easier for the two families involved. Plus, Christine and I love organization, so that was perfect for us as well. Still, there was so much that had to be done. Christine had already sent out her formal invitations, and RSVPs were sent back by the end of August.

I could not believe how fast the summer months had flown by. Christine had been extremely busy. The stress of her job on top of preparing for her big day was getting the best of her. She was trying to take care of too much all at the same time. I said, "Christine, do not be afraid to ask for help. If you don't ask, you don't get." That was something my daughter always had a very hard time doing. Once she asked for the help, her fiancé's family, my children, and I took some of the stress off of her. Christine and Garland appreciated that so much.

October 2014 had already arrived. I was in charge of decorating the wedding venue.

My mother, who was ninety-three years old at the time, was looking forward to attending. As my mother and I were talking on the telephone, she had some strong feelings that she wanted to share with me. In her own words, this is what she said:

My Mother: "Valerie, I feel that Christine's wedding is going to tell the story."

Me: "Really? Mom, what do you mean by that?"

My Mother: "Christine's wedding is going to show you exactly who is who."

Me: "Really?"

My Mother: "Yes. I feel that whoever is supposed to be at her wedding will be there. And, the ones that are not supposed to be there, for whatever reason, will not be there."

Me: "Really? That's something."

My Mother: "Ah ha. But, don't worry, Valerie, because the wedding is going to be beautiful."

Me: "That's good. What are you going to wear?"

My Mother: "I will be wearing a 'granny dress'."

Me: "A 'granny dress'. What do you mean by that?

My Mother: It's just a different type of dress than I normally wear, because this is you and your daughter's day.

Me: "Well, since the wedding ceremony is being held outside, I do hope the weather is good and that she has a beautiful day. Okay, Mom, I better get off the phone and do what I have to do for the wedding."

My Mother: "I love you."

Me: "I love you too, Mom."

The day before Christine and Garland's wedding, Christopher, Christel and I were so stressed out. We were running around like crazy doing last minute preparations. Plus, the day after the wedding, I was also having a get-together at my home with our close family and friends, since most of them lived out of town. So, everything needed to be taken care of all at the same time.

My children and I did not get any sleep at all that night. The morning of the wedding, my children and I could barely keep our eyes open, but we had to make the best of it. We still had so much to do that day. At 7:30 AM, my children and I rushed out of the house to go pick up the wedding cake and it looked absolutely beautiful. Then, we had to come back home and wait for Kail (my daughter's Man of Honor), so that he would be able to transport the wedding cake for me, and everything else that was needed, so that my children and I could decorate the hall.

After arriving at the hall, we all had to start the decorating process. Time was just moving too fast for all of us. After we had done what we had to do for the most part, we all rushed back home, got dressed, and came back to the venue in time for the wedding ceremony to take place. I had no idea how we were going to do all of that, but we did. We had to wait for our immediate family members to arrive, but once everyone was present, the announcement was made and the wedding ceremony began.

The ceremony took place on the outside grounds surrounding the lake. It was such a beautiful wedding ceremony and the weather was wonderful.

What was so unique for Christine and Garland's bridal party was that Christine had a Matron of Honor, a Man of Honor, and two bridesmaids. Garland had a Best Woman, a Best Man, and his brother was the

Groomsman. Garland's father was deceased so it was bittersweet, but there was a chair set in his honor on their special day.

Following the ceremony, pictures were taken. Then, everyone was able to enter into the beautiful, elegant silver, purple and white reception hall where we all enjoyed ourselves for the rest of the evening. My nephew, Jason, said at the hall, "Aunt Valerie, Christine's wedding was really nice." He said that he didn't know what to expect, but that he had a great time. Also, my cousin, Bernadette, told me that Christine's wedding was over the top and that she and her husband had a nice time.

I also felt good when Saycon's (one of the bridesmaids) mother, Deborah, came up to me and told me that Christine's wedding was just beautiful. She said that when she usually goes out, she doesn't stay out too long. She said the entire atmosphere of Christine's wedding felt so good and that she could not leave; she had to stay until the very end. That made me feel so good and I was happy that she was able to attend.

I was happy that everyone had a good time and enjoyed themselves. The bride and the groom were so happy.

Exit for the Bride and Groom

The night ended with everyone gathering outside. Andrea had us form two straight lines with our sparklers lit. She had me stand with my sparkler so when they came out I would be standing by the car waiting for them as they entered.

As the bride and groom walked fast down the middle, we all started shouting as they said their goodbyes to everyone. Christine came all the way down to where I was. She looked up at me before entering into the car and said, "Mom, I love you!" I really had to hold back my tears in that moment. As they drove away, I knew that she was well pleased with the way everything turned out.

What My Daughter, Christine Had to Endure

From the moment that Christine knew she was getting married, I just knew that her father would be more than happy to give his daughter away. As the time grew nearer and Christine was to soon be married, her father said that he may not be able to attend the wedding because he had to get some work done on his teeth— saying that he would not be able to smile. At that very moment, I could not believe that he would not show up for his daughter's special day. I also asked him if he would like to contribute something. You would have thought that I said something that was crazy. He did not even want to do that either. After that, Christine kept calling to speak with him and also to introduce her fiancé to him over the telephone. He was not having that either. The next thing Christine tried to do was to let Garland meet him in person. He had no intensions of making that happen.

So, I had a friend, Kenny—whom I have known since the spring of 1985 during our real estate school days— walk Christine down the aisle. At the time, Christine was only seven years old when they met. After we had moved to Atlanta, we kept in contact with him. Years passed and he also left New York City to make a better life for his daughter. Christine and I never even dreamed that, after Kenny had moved to Atlanta, he would be the one to walk her down the aisle.

Once Kenny was informed that Christine was getting married, the first thing that he asked was, "Am I walking Christine down the aisle?" I told him that I was trying to see what Christine's father was going to do first. He said, "If you need me to walk her down the aisle, that's no problem… I'll do it. Let me know." I said, "Okay." The time was getting near and we still did not hear back from Christine's father.

We continued calling, but he never even had the decency to respond back to either of us. Christine was feeling so bad that she cried for days wondering what the outcome was going to be. And, still we never heard a response back. I was so mad.

When I called Kenny again, he said, "Am I in?" I told him, "Yes." He was so happy! I told him that Christine's father never even acknowledged her wedding. Kenny said, "She does not deserve that. It's his loss." I felt so relieved. Kenny always wanted to be that special father figure to Christine. God gave Christine that gift of love that she received from Kenny on her wedding day. He was the one that was supposed to walk my daughter down the aisle. And, he did it so willingly and happily. Christine and I both knew that Kenny was more like a father to her than her own father was. Plus, Christine always felt close to Kenny.

Christine talked about the memories that she shared with Kenny as a young child growing up: She said that Kenny was the first person to show her how to use a knife and fork to cut her food; he attended her dance recitals in New York, as well as her performances in Atlanta. She said that she appreciated that big red bike he purchased for her, but still have not learned to ride yet. Those were just a few special memories in Christine's life that she could never forget.

Who would have known, after all of those years since we have known Kenny, that on October 18, 2014 he would be the one giving Christine away? That was such a special moment in Christine's life and one she will treasure forever.

A Gathering at My Home

That very next day, I was so happy that family and friends gathered at my home to continue the celebration of Christine and Garland's wedding weekend. It was so nice seeing everyone, but the time went by too fast.

With everything I had gone through during that particular time, I was so happy that my lupus did not flare-up on me at all. I was very pleased that everything turned out so well.

Lupus Clinic Appointment - 11/11/14

The morning of November 11, 2014, I had an appointment at the Lupus Clinic. After my blood pressure was checked, it was found to be a little high. Therefore, the doctor felt that it was time to put me on a 25 mg tablet of Hydrochlorothiazide, but only as needed. That meant that I had to check my blood pressure daily. I was advised to take: one 300 mg tablet of Allopurinol daily, one 10 mg tablet of Amlodipine Besylate daily, one 0.6 mg tablet of Colcrys as needed, and one 100 mg tablet of Losartan Potassium daily.

An Ending to a New Year

During the Thanksgiving and Christmas holiday, I was home celebrating nicely with my family. When New Year's Eve came, it was brought in by relaxing, eating, and watching television with my two children, Christopher and Christel. They never seem to enjoy all the fuss over New Year's Eve. They always said, "It's just another New Year's Eve to us." For me, it was a blessing to still be alive.

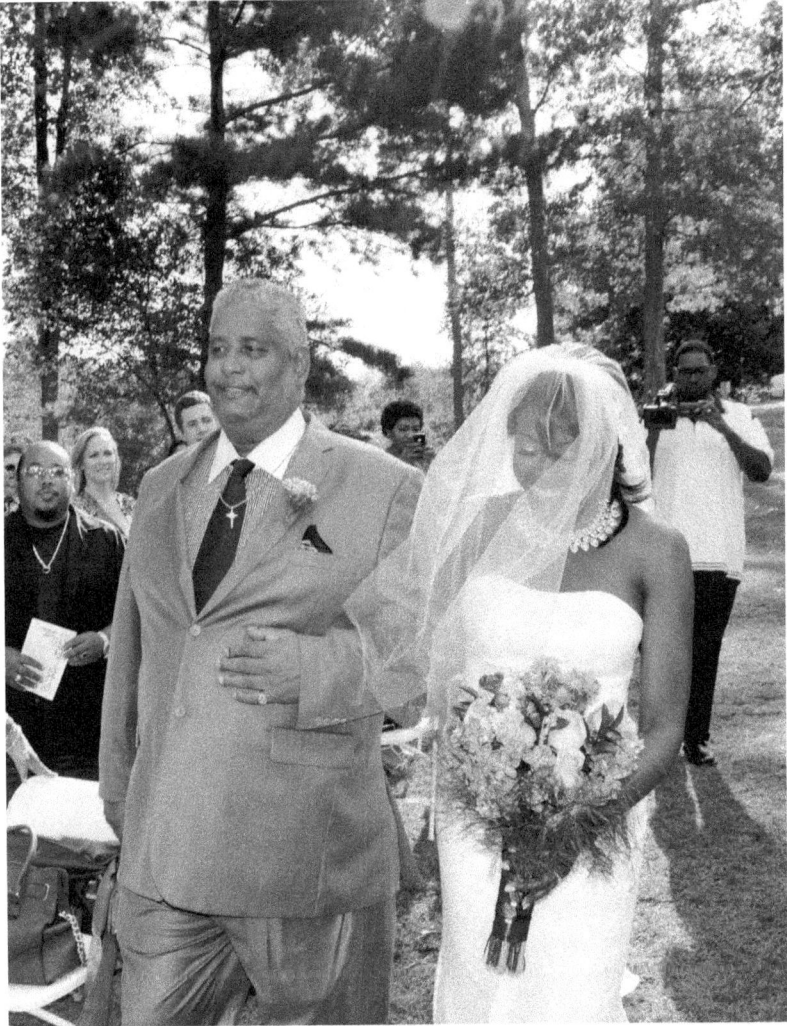

My Daughter's Wedding Day - October 18, 2014.
Kenny giving my daughter, Christine away.

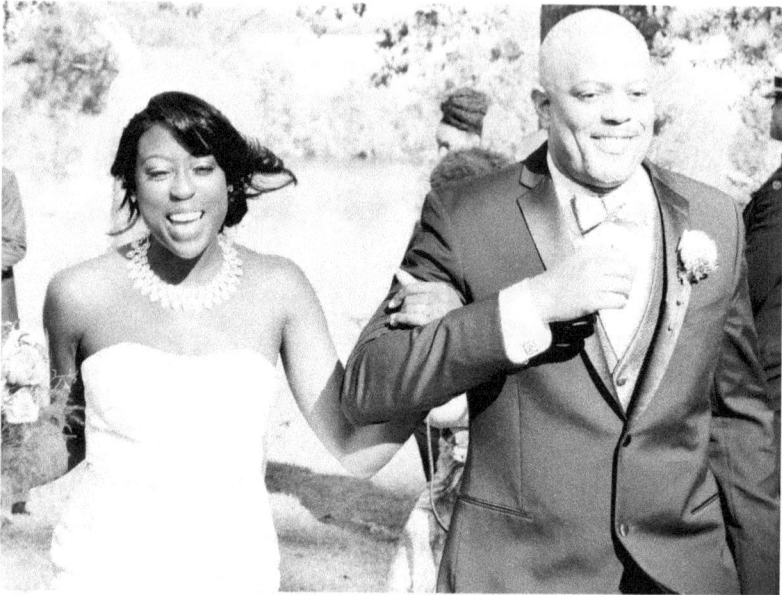

Officially husband and wife.
Christine and Garland E Raiford, III

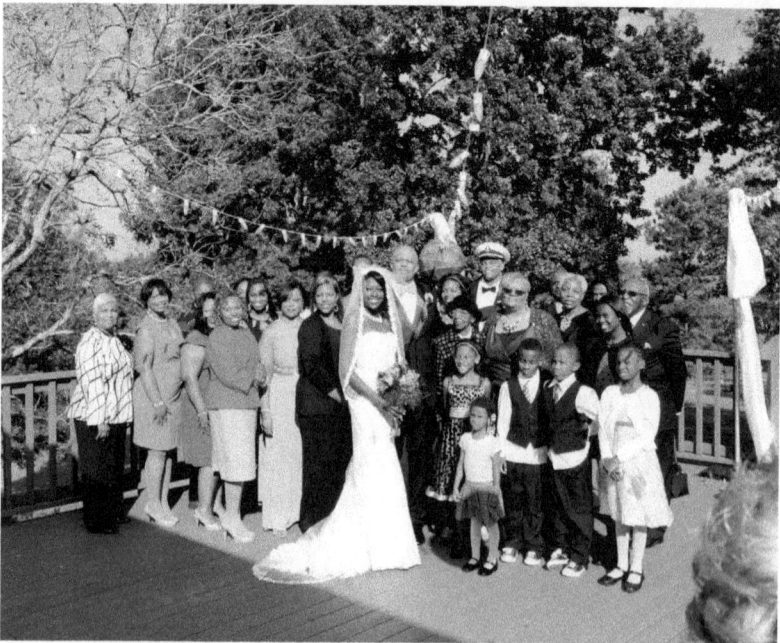

A group picture of the groom's family members.

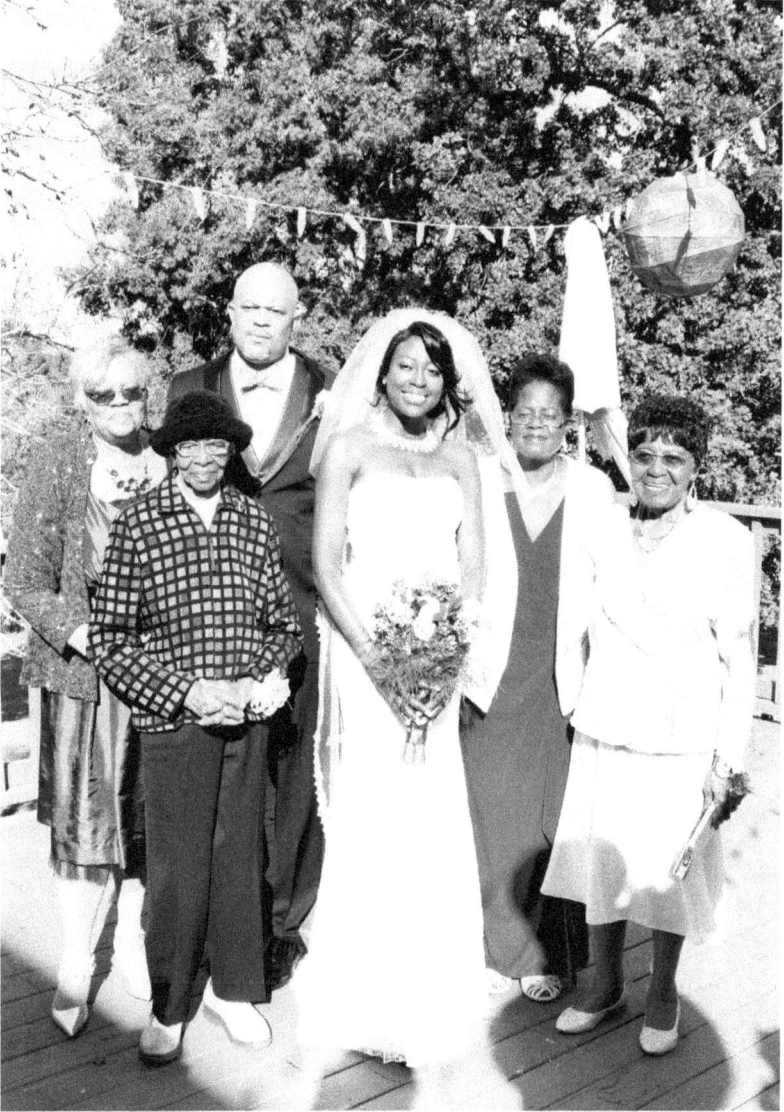

Our picture was taken with the bride and groom.
Left side: Groom's mother and his grandmother.
Right side: My mother and I.

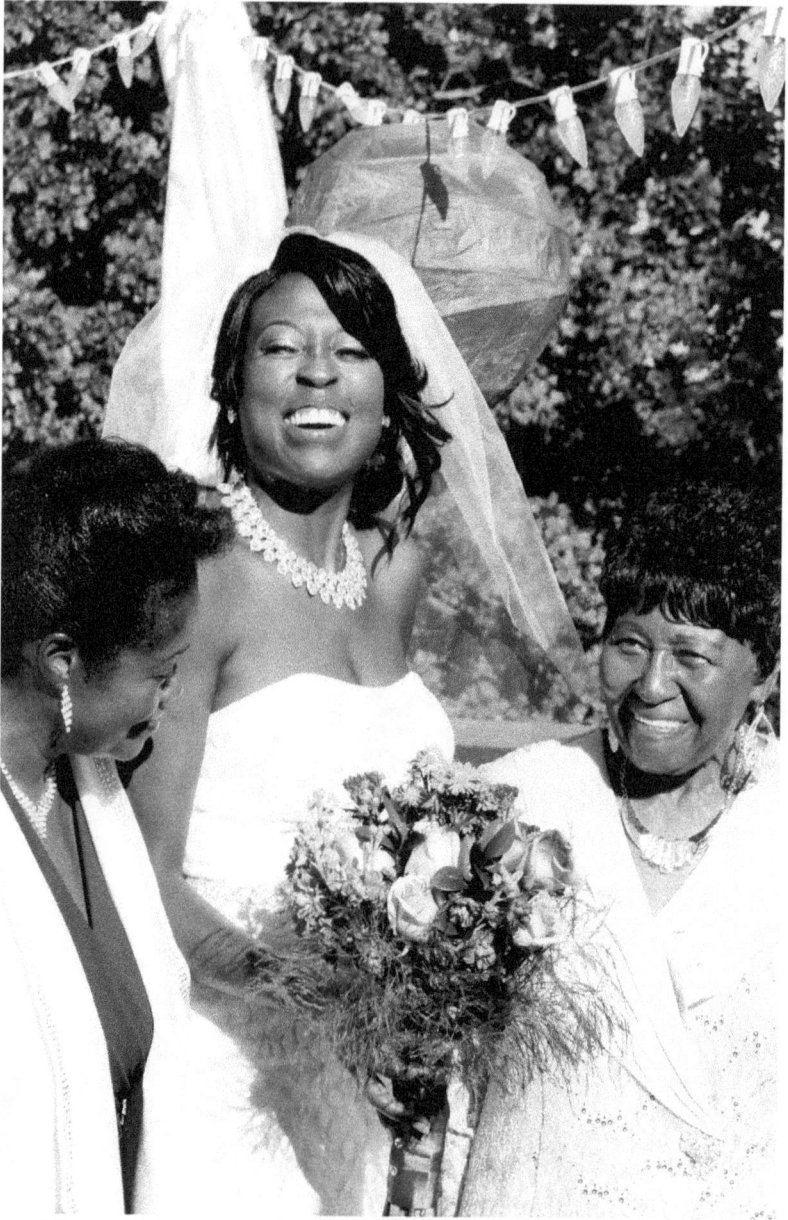

Me, my daughter, and my mother, sharing a laughing moment together.

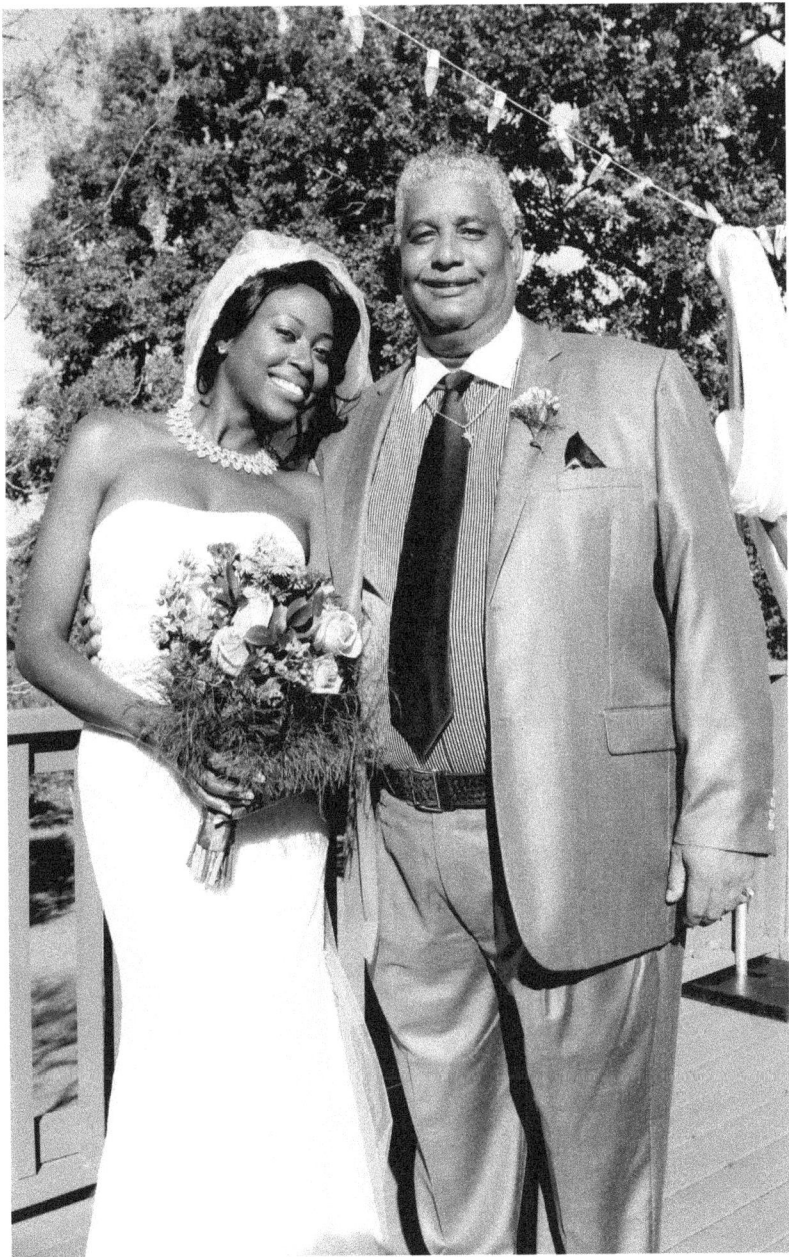

My daughter, Christine and Kenny.

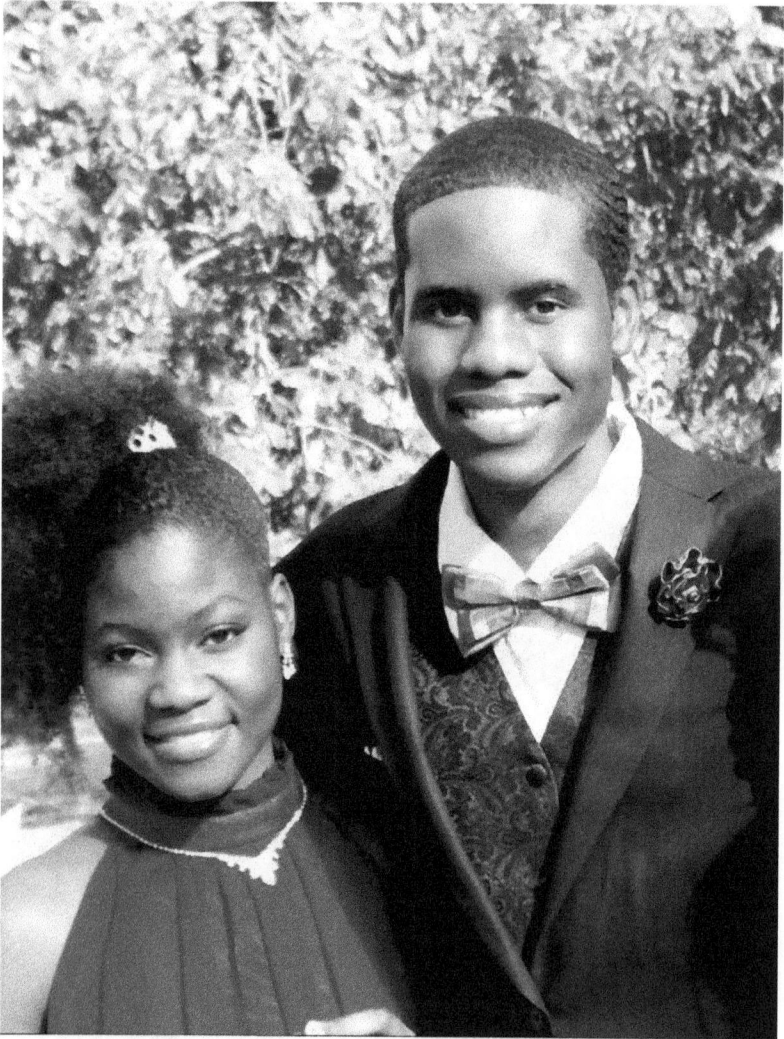

My youngest daughter, Christel and my son, Christopher.

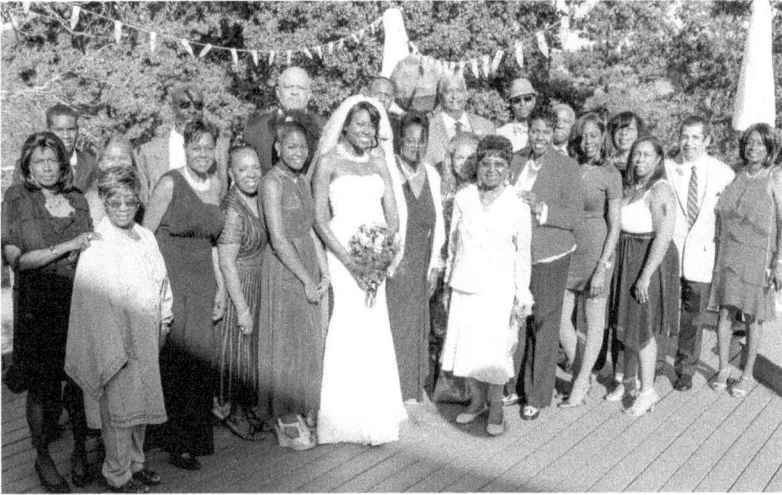

A group picture taken of my family members.

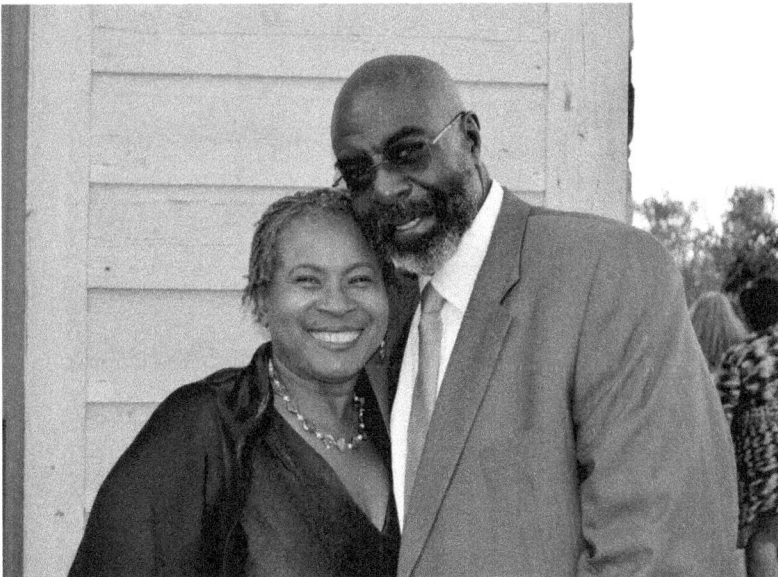

My cousin Marcus and his wife Bernalyn.

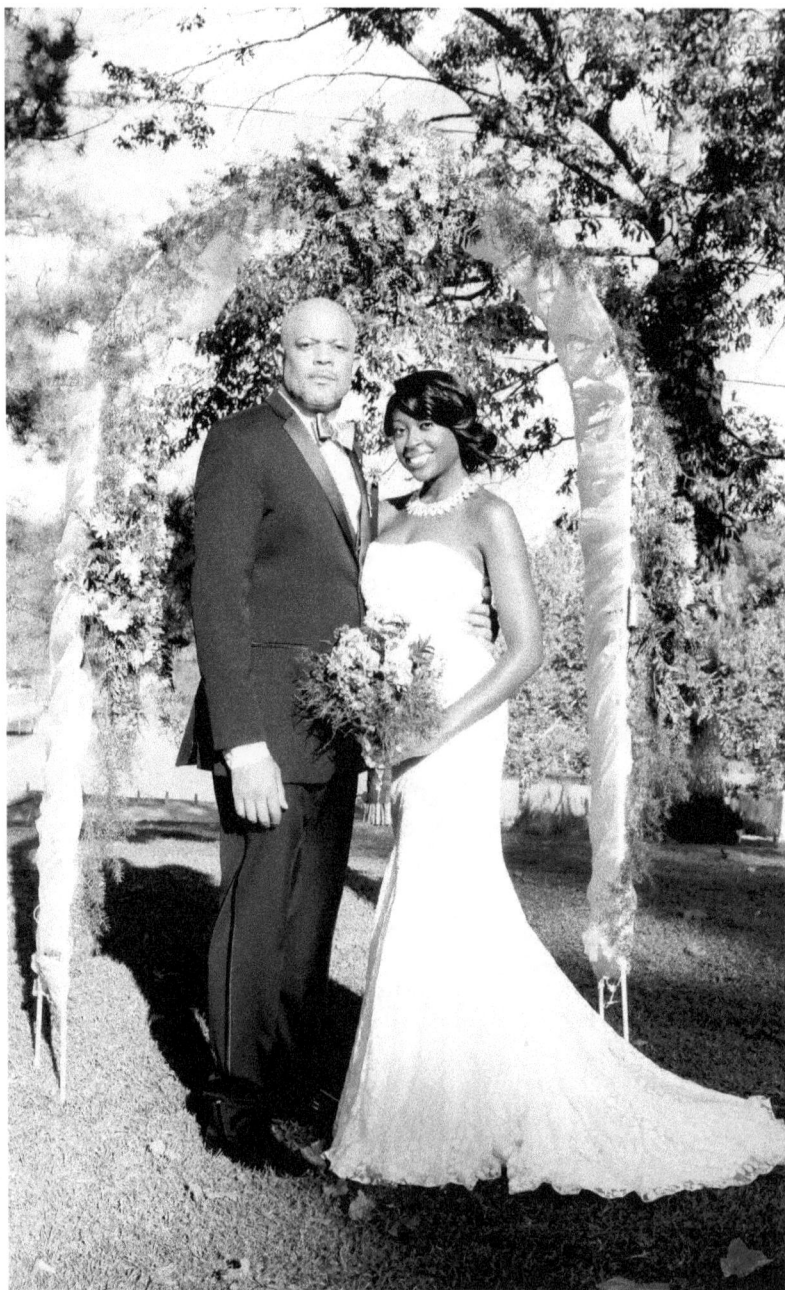

Christine and Garland E. Raiford, III

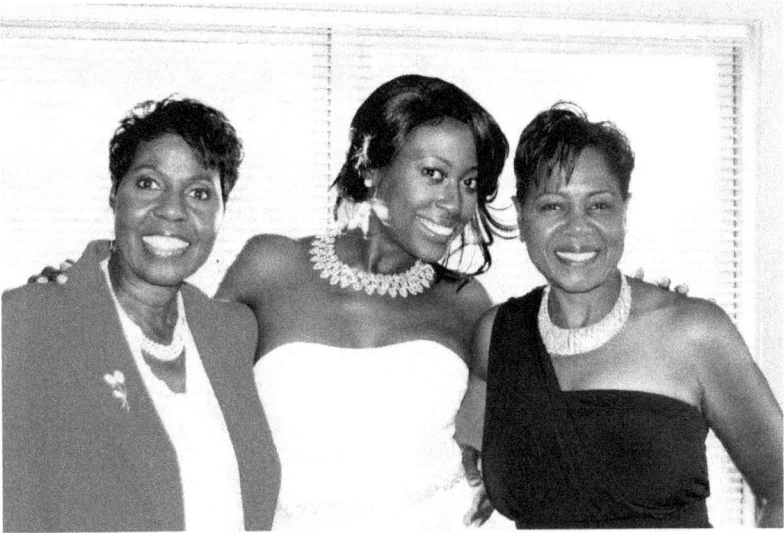

My daughter, and my two sisters.
Left side: Claudette
Right side: Vanessa

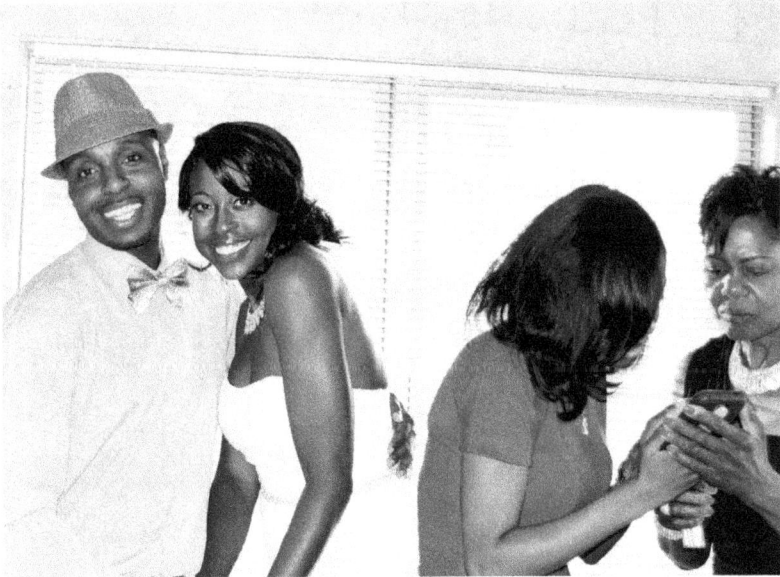

Left to right: My nephew, Jason, my daughter, Christine, my niece
Melissa, and my sister, Vanessa.

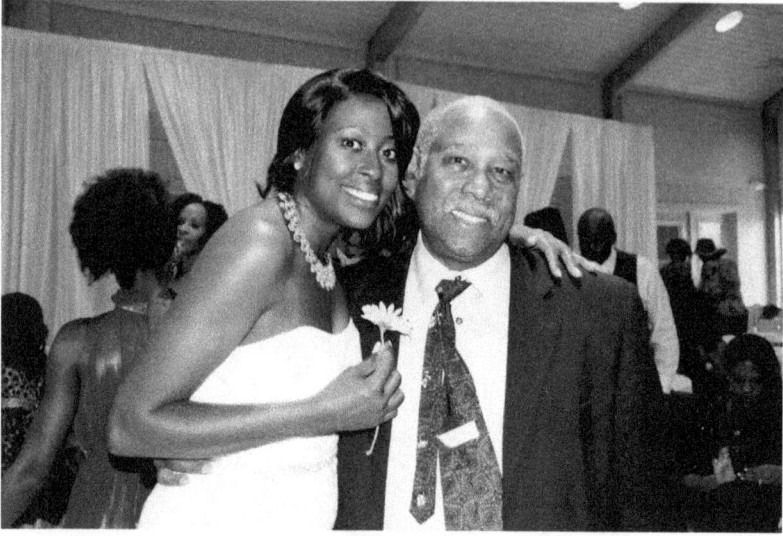

My daughter, and our cousin Leonard.

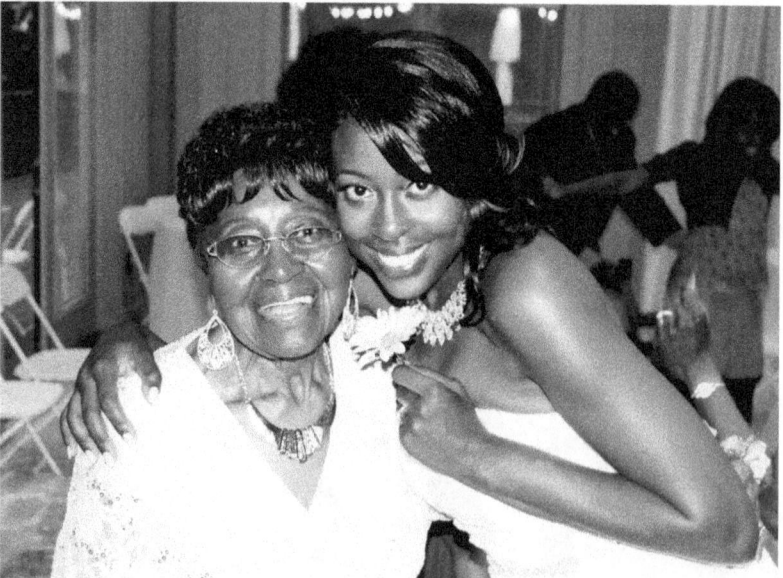

My mother, and my daughter.

An Exit for the Bride and Groom.
Everyone gathered outside with their sparklers.

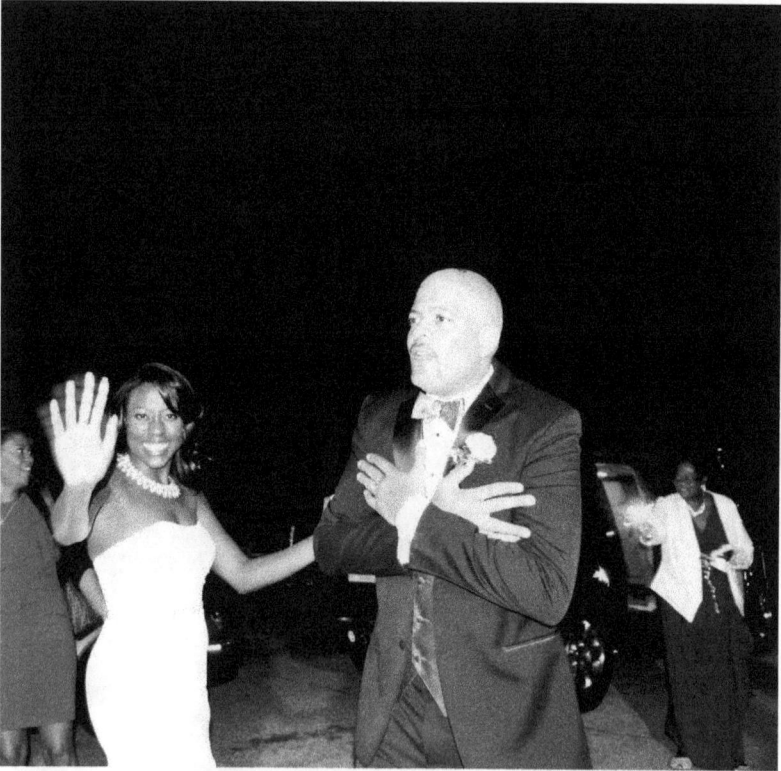

Christine and Garland were leaving.
(Picture of me in the background on the right).

CONCLUSION

My lupus journey has taken you through the most vulnerable time in my life. I shared my up and down moments, as well as my lupus flare-ups and remission cycles that repeated themselves at any given time during the course of my illness. Lupus does not always reappear in the exact same way that it last occurred. Faith, courage, and positive energy, gives me the strength to keep moving forward.

Currently, I am still battling lupus, but my health has been steadily improving. As I reminisce about all the things that I have been through, I hope that my story can be an inspiration to lupus patients and to those who also may be suffering with some type of illness.

I continue to live a fulfilled life, receiving medical treatment by a caring team of doctors at Grady Memorial Hospital. This was my story; this was

LUPUS: The Battle Within.

TO MY READERS

I would like to take this opportunity to thank each and every one of you, who have decided to pick up and read my lupus story. I have taken you through my most precious, private, and most intimate moments of my life.

I hope this book has enlightened you to the challenges one may face, despite the odds. I know that lupus will always be my constant battle and my never-ending journey.

I thank God each and every day for the gifts that I have been given and the strength to keep moving forward. I hope that this book can help give you that same kind of strength.

ACKNOWLEDGEMENTS

I would like to thank the following people who have made my book possible:

Christine Lauren Horn Raiford, my daughter: I love you and thank you so much for what you have done for me. This book would not have even been possible without the love, support, and encouragement that you have given me to write my "lupus" story.

Christopher Samuel Bethune, my son: I love you and thank you so much for your hard work and devotion to this project. I am so grateful for the wonderful job you have done.

Christel Diamond Bethune, my daughter: I love you and thank you for understanding my long nights at the computer, and for giving me your input and honest opinion when it was needed.

Lillian Colley, my mother: I love you and thank you so much for the advice you have given, by letting me know that it was definitely okay to show pictures of how lupus has affected me.

Dr. Christine Lawrence and Dr. Betty Diamond: Thank you so much for being there to help me when I was very young and extremely ill. I also thank you for being such caring doctors to me all of these years. My life would not have been the same without you. I am also grateful that I was able to share those experiences in my book.

ABOUT THE AUTHOR

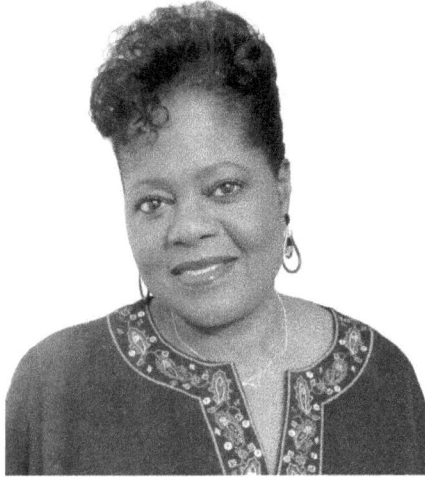

Valerie Horn was born and raised in New York City. She worked as a legal secretary for over seventeen years, as well as pursuing a career in real estate. Valerie never let her lupus define her and worked diligently to maintain her goals in life. In 1992, Valerie relocated to Atlanta, Georgia. Valerie is a single parent of three, who has instilled in her children the value of a good education, to be the best that they can be, and encouraged them to always follow their dreams.

Valerie's experience with lupus, from her flare-ups and remission cycles, to all of the diagnoses she has received, has certainly not been easy. She has been coping with this incurable disease for many years and refuses to let it get the best of her. From being a very strong and courageous woman, she has overcome a tremendous amount of obstacles in her life. Valerie is an active participant in the GOAL (Georgians Organized Against

Lupus) study project by Emory University's Division of Rheumatology. She attends lupus support group meetings, as well as keeping abreast of all the information given from the Lupus Foundation of America.

Valerie's greatest accomplishment is her first book, "Lupus: The Battle Within." She shares her most intimate life story battling lupus from childhood to adulthood, while staying positive, and living her life to the fullest. In her spare time, she enjoys writing, as well as her passion for painting, masonry work, and interior decorating. Valerie has many artistic talents. Her love of the beautiful outdoors includes gardening and nature, which always seems to fulfill her.

Valerie's journey, "Lupus: The Battle Within,"
can also be found at her website at
www.valeriehorn.com.

ABOUT THE ILLUSTRATOR

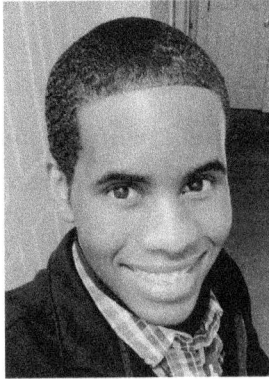

Christopher Bethune is an Illustrator and Graphic Designer who resides in Atlanta, Georgia. During his childhood years, art was always a passion of his. He became very influenced in Japanese art culture, as well as storytelling, at a very young age. Since Christopher began kindergarten, and all the way into his senior year in high school, he decided to take his skills to the next level. Christopher Bethune attended The Art Institute of Atlanta and majored in Illustration and Design. After four years in college, he received his Bachelor's Degree in Fine Arts, as well as winning "Best in Show" for Illustration and Design during the summer of 2013. After his biggest accomplishment, he was fortunate enough to work for Georgia Tech as a Digital Designer: designing posters, animations, business cards, as well as other projects for different clients.

Christopher's mother, Valerie Horn, decided that she

wanted to write a book about her life and her struggles battling lupus. Christopher was excited to be a part of this project, not only because he was her son, but to prove to himself that he was also a jack-of-all-trades.

Christopher Bethune states: *"It has been an honor and a privilege to do a project for someone so special. In life, we always want to know what our purpose is. I can truly say that I have found it. I have seen my mother struggle through both the good times and the bad, so I already know her story. For the people who don't, then this book "Lupus: The Battle Within," will take you on a journey—showing one woman beating against all odds. Mom, thank you so much for always believing in me, and pushing me, to be the best person I can be. I love you!"*

To see Christopher Bethune's projects, please visit www.christopherbethune.artworkfolio.com.

A NOTE FROM THE EDITOR

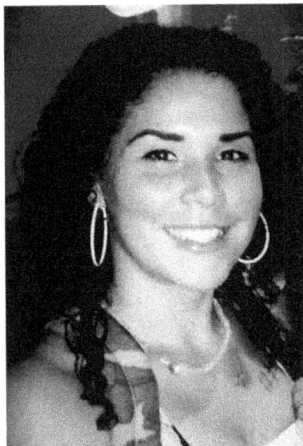

Writing a book is a very vulnerable act. You are essentially laying your heart out on these pages and sending it out into the world. It takes a tremendous amount of courage and a healthy dose of self-worth to share your story with others. The journey that Valerie has chosen to share with us is one of considerable pain and suffering, but also one of considerable love and support from the people that matter most. If nothing else touches you about her story, I hope that you can at least recognize the blessings in your own life and truly appreciate the struggle that Valerie has overcome. She has taken an incurable disease and turned it into a topic of inspiration; sharing with readers that, not only can you live with lupus, you can thrive with it. Life is what you make it and, looking back, Valerie did not let her illness define her. She used it as the catalyst to ignite all of the beautiful things she has accomplished in life—from her career to her children and beyond. For those who are also living with lupus, and other health obstacles, please take Valerie's story to heart; and let it be a reminder to you that you can overcome absolutely anything with a positive attitude and people that love you.

Valerie—I sincerely congratulate you on not only setting this goal for yourself, but for accomplishing it as well. I wish you nothing but success and good health! It has been an honor to be a part of this journey with you. Thank you.

Courtney Lindemann